AF531310

World Trade Organisation and Food Security

World Trade Organisation and Food Security

By

Dr. M. Lakshmi Narasaiah
M.A., Ph.D.
Professor of Economics,
Coordinator, Department of M.B.A.
Sri Krishnadevaraya University Post-graduate Centre,
Kurnool–518 002
Andhra Pradesh (India)

DISCOVERY PUBLISHING HOUSE
NEW DELHI

First Published–2005

ISBN: 81-7141-940-2

Published by:

DISCOVERY PUBLISHING HOUSE

4831/24, Prahlad Street, Ansari Road, Darya Ganj
New Delhi–110 002 (India)
Phone: 23279245, • Fax: 91-11-23253475
e-mail: dphtemp@indiatimes.com

Printed at:
Amit Enterprises, Delhi

Preface

The reason why trade has such a vital part to play in building peace is because it means lowering barriers—not only to goods and services but among nations and peoples. The elimination of barriers creates interdependence and interdependence creates solidarity. The history of the last fifty years has shown us all the undeniable benefits of lowering trade barriers and opening economies.

Clearly every region has its own characteristics, and it would be wrong to imagine that the same blueprint can apply everywhere and in the same way. Any region which way for thousands of years at the crossroads of world trade should regain its place in the centre, because doing so will help build peace as well as prosperity. This is why the numerous applications for accession to the WTO from various countries are so significant. The first is through regionalism. There are several efforts at regional trade and economic initiatives among countries, and that such initiatives will be encouraged to reduce positive results. Regional initiatives are important because they can help countries at a comparable level of development to move relatively quickly in opening their economies and in deepening their interdependence.

However, the rapid advance of global economic integration means that while regional initiatives remain important, they are not sufficient by themselves to address successfully the new perspectives of the international economy. That is why there is a need for second track, which is the rule-based multilateral system. And that is why the multilateral system is of fundamental importance to the economic prosperity of any region.

As the first major international institution to be created in the post-Cold War era, the WTO offers a promise of the kind of global economic architecture which need in the coming decades. Its culture is firmly rooted in the tradition of consensus-building and cooperation among sovereign countries. And the WTO embodies rights and obligations negotiated by consensus, approved and ratified by each government and each Parliament, and they are enforceable, not through the crude exercise of economic power, but through the rule of law. The alternative would be a power-based system—who would want to chose this option?

But most importantly, the WTO is an organisation which brings all countries—from all corners of the world and from all levels of development—together as equals. There is no weighted voting, no exclusive clubs, no inner and outer circles. Developing countries representing 80% of constituency sit as equals with industrialised countries to write the rules of a shared trading system.

This new unity of developing and developed countries inside a single system will be credited as the greatest achievement of the multilateral system. But this unity is still fragile: We cannot allow it to be broken: This is why, in preparing the agenda of the first Ministerial meeting in Singapore, have recognised the particular difficult task facing developing countries in implementing the Uruguay Round commitments. They have also acknowledged the challenges they face in contemplating the necessary work programme.

The integration of developing countries as equal partners in the multilateral system is one of the most important challenges in shaping the economic order of the 21st century. This is a shared responsibility of developed and developing countries alike. There is no rational alternative to this objective. The evolution of the global economy makes that clear.

Now there is a need to work together as equal partners to ensure the full integration, and all other developing and transition economies, into the global economy and the rule-based multilateral trading system. In conjunction with this there is a need to encourage, notably the growth of regional economic cooperation. The alternative is a vicious circle where economic isolation feeds greater political instability which in turn leads to greater economic isolation. The road to a lasting peace in the world begins, not ends, with economic integration and interdependence. Taking this message to heart will help build a future where it is goods, services, and investment that cross borders—not missiles and soldiers.

Dr. M. Lakshmi Narasaiah

Contents

1

World Trade–The Next Challenge

On 15 December 1993 the world changed. My be not as dramatically as the moment when the Berlin Wall fell, but then unlike that very necessary demolition job, the success of the Uruguay Round was a work of construction. Like the destruction of the wall, though, its effects will be profound and lasting ones felt far beyond its immediate context. It will be seen as a defining moment in modern history.

The importance of the Round can be seen in terms of boost it gives to job creation; to development; to investment; to economic reform; to the rule of law and in many other ways besides. All of these benefits are real and important. But the true value of the whole is much, much more than the sum of these parts.

Put simply, governments came to the conclusion that the notion of a new world order was not merely attractive but absolutely vital; that the reality of the global market–whatever ambitions some of them may retain for regional Integration–required a level of multilateral cooperation never before attempted.

No Losers in The Round

It has created a revolutionary framework for economic, legal and political cooperation. But now turn to the immediate results of the Round. Seeing them as a profit and loss account or a scorecard of winners and losers is to see them in static terms, as one-off conclusions with finite effects. This misses the point completely.

Every nation now needs an effective trading system, but especially so that small and poor. They have it. Everyone will also gain from the huge package of market access results even if they did not get every concession they were seeking from trading partners—it is the biggest market access deal ever negotiated.

However, the essence of the Uruguay Round's achievements is that they are dynamic. The new agreements, the new rules and structures it sets up—all mean a commitment to a continuing process of cooperation and reform of which the agreement in December was only the beginning.

Maintaining the liberalizing momentum will call for continuing effort and vigilance by participating countries. But now their energy can be focused through the Round's greatest innovation; the new World Trade Organisation (WTO) in place of the improvised basis on which the GATT has operated for 45 years, trade will now have a permanent forum appropriate to its importance in the world economy.

Technically speaking, the WTO will oversee the implementation of the Round's results, administer all the agreements in goods, services and intellectual property, and manage the unified dispute settlement system. But beyond these administrative functions, it will raise the political profile of trade a profile which has already been lifted greatly by the Uruguay Round. The WTO will have regular instead of occasional—direct Ministerial involvement. It will have a clear mandate to act as a forum for further trade negotiations. Most of all it will complete the transition from a trading system which largely restricted itself to policies at the border to one which also covers most aspects of domestic policy-making affecting international competition in goods and services, as well as investment.

Through the WTO, the Round will change the way the world economy is shaped. But it is not the final victory over protectionism and unilateralism. Any premature rejoicing would have quickly been cut short by the evidence since 15 December that major economic powers are still ready to take the unilateral approach to trade problems. Arguments for protectionism based on the alleged threat of low-cost competition to production and jobs will not just fade away because the Round is a success. The seductive appeal of "beggar-thy-neighbour" policies is highlighted by the seemingly greater vigour of the lobbies for protectionism than the advocates of open markets.

These dangers—and the speed with which they have resurfaced—make the achievement of the Uruguay Round all the more important, and its successful implementation all the more urgent. Implementation requires more than mutual backslapping about what we have achieved. It requires now that the US, EU and Japan, in particular, rapidly obtain final authority to ratify and also take a lead in providing the WTO with the means to fulfill its mandate.

The success of the Round has come at a time when it is even more vitally needed than anyone could have guessed when it was launched in 1986. Old structures and alignments have been turned inside out in trade as in every other area of international relations. We face a world of change and challenge, in which the reinforced trading system will be a primary source of stability and security.

The developing countries including India have become enthusiastic supporters of the multilateral trading system and the Uruguay Round every if all their demands were not met by industrial countries. The reasons lie in the changing economic policies of many developing countries and the clearer appreciation of the value of the GATT system that has grown along with these changes.

The challenge of new issues in world trade will be a major one for the WTO. The new organisation has to consider issues such as the links between trade and the environment, international competition policy, trade and investment, and trade and labour standards. To say a few words about trade and the environment since it is one area in which GATT member countries have committed themselves already to a comprehensive new work programme. They decided on 15 December, in conjunction with the adoption of the results of the Uruguay Round negotiations, to draw up a work programme on trade and environment by the Ministerial meeting in Marrakesh. Environmental policy-making is one of the most rapidly evolving areas of national and international policy-making, and it is entirely appropriate that emphasis should be placed now in GATT/WTO on ensuring better policy coordination and multilateral cooperation over the linkages between trade and environment.

Permanent Negotiations

The Uruguay Round may well be the last of its kind, but this in no way means the end of multilateral trade negotiations. On the contrary, it means they become a permanent event. Ad hoc negotiating rounds were necessary mainly because the GATT lacked the mandate or the institutional basis to operate the multilateral system to the full on a continuous basis. Between rounds the GATT has tended to lose momentum, often at the very times when it was essential to make the most of the liberalising impulse. This has allowed protectionism and unilateralism to recover and regroup and meant that each round has to start by regaining lost ground.

The positive results of the Uruguay Round will redefine much more than assumptions about trade. If they are exploited with the same determination, courage and commitment that went into concluding the Round, they should mean nothing less than a new start for sustainable growth and a new system of collective economic security for the world.

But if the trading system is now up to the job of supporting multilateral cooperation on such a wide scale, do the other structures of economic cooperation still meet the bill? The establishment of the WTO will put trade and investment on a par—perhaps rather in advance—of cooperation in monetary and financial areas. The WTO will stand alongside its original Bretton Woods sisters, the IMF and the World Bank. The three institutions must learn to work together even more effectively and closely. For example, rather than each body conducting separate reviews of country policies, is there not a case to be made for a more integrated approach on country reviews? But that does not, on its own, add up to effective multilateral economic cooperation. The question really has to be asked seriously: are the G7, the OECD, the regional groupings adequate to provide that cooperation?

It is the next challenge of international economic leadership—the challenge of translating the common interest in global growth into a practical and effective mechanism for solving our common economic problems together. So, the Ministers meeting in Marrakesh is an historic event which will establish the World Trade Organisation and put in place the new multilateral trading system, they will be making not an end, but a beginning.

2

International Trade with the Consumer's Money

When trade policies are discussed nationally or internationally people as consumers are largely forgotten. Despite their numbers, they do not carry the weight that producers and other lobbies command. Individually, consumers are seldom informed about how the availability, quality, price and choice of the hundreds of items which they buy in the shops each year are affected by trade policy decisions. If they know how much of their household budgets are determined by decisions to protect individual industries and for how little effect they might be shocked.

Equally, when it is debated publicly, the benefits that would fall to the consumer are usually ignored. This brief study is an attempt to put the consumer interest squarely in the public arena.

How Do Government Decisions on Trade Affect the Consumer?

Virtually all-protective policies mean higher prices for the consumer. And if it is not a consumer who pays, it will be domestic producer. These are some of the main actions taken by national authorities.

Governments frequently and for the most part, legally raise revenue and protect domestic industries by imposing duties on imported products. If a product has a 25 per cent tariff, the price in the shop will normally be 25 per cent more than its price at the port or airport.

Global quotas and other numerical limits on imports are sometimes legal sometimes not. Either way the intention is to restrict access to the market in such a away that domestic producers of the same product can raise their prices without being forced out of business through lack of competitiveness. Quotas are frequently preferred by those demanding protection because the impact on prices is less obvious than with a tariff. Once again, prices go up in the shops and limits may be so narrow that goods disappear from the shelves altogether.

Voluntary export restraints are quotas of an even more costly kind for the importing country. They allow foreign suppliers to charge higher prices than would be possible under a tariff or normal quota. By "bribing" the exporter this way, opposition to the protection is reduced.

Subsidies are sometimes paid to domestic producers to help them compete with import competition by keeping their costs artificially low. This keeps prices down. Unfortunately, the consumer as a tax payer ends up paying for the subsidy. In so doing, he is prevented from keeping more of his income to spend on other goods, which may be produced by more efficient industries. One thing is sure once industries get used to subsidies, it is very hard to wean then away.

Rules permit governments to impose extra duties on imports where products are shown to be dumped (sold below the normal price in the exporting country) or subsidised, and where the effect of dumping or subsidisation is demonstrated to damage the corresponding domestic industry. While these duties may be justified, they nevertheless always serve to raise the price for consumers to knock products completely out of the market. Yet very few, if any, countries give much weight to consumer interest when deciding whether to impose such penalty duties. And their use had grown disturbingly in recent years.

Governments usually impose standards of safety, quality, public health and environmental protection for good reasons often in the interests of consumers. Sometimes, however, the standards and the procedures which enforce them are no more than hidden protection for domestic producers. In imposing unnecessary measures on imports, governments penalize consumers through higher prices and the non-availability of goods.

Protection tends to be loaded towards the products which are essentials for any family. Consequently, since the essential command the biggest proportion of the household budgets of poor families, protection acts as a regressive tax.

Clothing is a good example. The multifibre arrangement acts on low-cost products, raising prices and restricting availability, meanwhile up-market goods are seldom affected. Moreover, for the poor consumer, the effect is further exaggerated. Foreign producers will tend to export higher quality end, therefore, more expensive goods, in order to maximize their profits from the quota. This quality upgrading effect not only reduces disproportionately the supply of lower-priced clothing, but may also affect the supply of children's clothing.

Consumers have enjoyed an enormous growth in the range and quality of products in their shops as a result of the multi-lateral training system. Many fruit and vegetables are available even out of season throughout the year. Exotic foods, never seen just ten or twenty years ago, are now commonly found on super-market selves. Cut flowers are being transported fresh by cargo plane daily from one country to the other. The range and sophi-stication of domestic electronic products would have been unimagi-nable had their development not been spurred by the availability of a global market.

Household Costs are Not the Only Consumer Cost which go Up

Many industries are also consumers of imported goods. Manufacturers can depend on cheaper and better products from overseas in order to maintain their own competitiveness in their domestic market and, especially, in their export markets.

The best example is steel. Many companies require either specialty steel or basic steel products at the lowest possible prices. Unfortunately, because of export restraints, formal quotas, ant-dumping and countervailing duties and high tariffs. Sometimes they cannot even find the precise type or quality of steel they need. They are, therefore, put at a huge competitive disadvantage.

Semi-conductors and other electronic components are also subject to this self defeating form of protection. Just as the price of steel puts up the price of automobiles, so high tariffs, anti-dumping duties and quotas on electronic components puts up the prices of video recorders, personal computers and other advanced consumer electronic products. Meanwhile foreign competitors continue to buy their semi-conductor inputs at world market prices.

But is One of the Prices a Lowering of Public Health and Safety Standards?

It has been suggested that some measures to ensure safe good for consumers and to prevent the spread of pests of diseases among animals and plants do not amount to unjustified barriers to trade.

The first point is that if there is some justification for them, these measures—even if they restrict trade—are completely permissable. The main objective is to make them transparent, to discourage arbitrary decision-making and discrimination and to minimize any restriction on trade.

The second point is that would encourage governments to establish measures consistent with international standards and guidelines. This is important because it could mean a general raising of standards: in many areas even advanced industrial countries do not meet international standards on food safety.

Third, the governments has to impose more stringent standards than those agreed internationally. The only condition is that a government so doing might, if challenged, be required to show scientific evidence or some kind of risk assessment to support the measure.

It should also be noted that with the reduction of agricultural subsidies which encourage unlimited production (those supporting farmers' income directly will still be permitted) consumers should see more products produced by less chemical intensive farming methods in the shops.

3

Trading Towards Peace

The reason why trade has such a vital part to play in building peace is because it means lowering barriers—not only to goods and services but among nations and peoples. The elimination of barriers creates interdependence and interdependence creates solidarity. The history of the last fifty years has shown us all the undeniable benefits of lowering trade barriers and opening economies.

Clearly every region has its own characteristics, and it would be wrong to imagine that the same blueprint can apply everywhere and in the same way. Any region which was for thousands of years at the crossroads of world trade should regain its place in the centre, because doing so will help build peace as well as prosperity. This is why the numerous applications for accession to the WTO from various countries are so significant. The first is through regionalism. There are several efforts at regional trade and economic initiatives among countries, and that such initiatives will be encouraged to reduce positive results. Regional initiatives are important because they can help countries at a comparable level of development to move relatively quickly in opening their economies and in deepening their interdependence.

However, the rapid advance of global economic integration means that while regional initiatives remain important, they are not sufficient by themselves to address successfully the new perspectives of the international economy. That is why there is a need for second track, which is the rule-based multilateral system. And that is why the multilateral system is of fundamental importance to the economic prosperity of any region.

As the first major international institution to be created in the post-Cold War era, the WTO offers a promise of the kind of global economic architecture which need in the coming decades. Its culture is firmly rooted in the tradition of consensus-building and cooperation among sovereign countries. And the WTO embodies rights and obligations negotiated by consensus, approved and ratified by each government and each Parliament, and they are enforceable, not through the crude exercise of economic power, but through the rule of law. The alternative would be a power-based system—who would want to chose this option ?

But most importantly, the WTO is an organisation which brings all countries—from all corners of the world and from all levels of development—together as equals. There is no weighted voting, no exclusive clubs, no inner and outer circles. Developing countries representing 80% of constituency sit as equals with industrialised countries to write the rules of a shared trading system.

This new unity of developing and developed countries inside a single system will be credited as the greatest achievement of the multilateral system. But this unity is still fragile: We cannot allow it to be broken: This is why, in preparing the agenda of the first Ministerial meeting in Singapore, have recognised the particular difficult task facing developing countries in implementing the Uruguay Round commitments. They have also acknowledged the challenges they face in contemplating the necessary work programme.

The integration of developing countries as equal partners in the multilateral system is one of the most important challenges in shaping the economic order of the 21st century. This is a shared responsibility of developed and developing countries alike. There is no rational alternative to this objective. The evolution of the global economy makes that clear.

Now there is a need to work together as equal partners to ensure the full integration, and all other developing and transition economies, into the global economy and the rule-based multilateral trading system. In conjunction with this there is a need to encourage, notably the growth of regional economic cooperation. The alternative is a vicious circle where economic isolation feeds greater political instability which in turn leads to greater economic isolation. The road to a lasting peace in the world begins, not ends, with economic integration and interdependence. Taking this message to heart will help build a future where it is goods, services, and investment that cross borders—not missiles and soldiers.

4

Free Trade as Peacemaker:

The Benefits of an Open World Trading System

Globalisation by free trade according to the principles of the World Trade Organisation (WTO) offers the only realistic opportunity to integrate the world peacefully and in time to prevent a major disaster. The primacy of the economy over politics is the most important vehicle for a successful world domestic policy.

Since Adam Smith, traditional economic theory has on principle been well-disposed towards free trade. Free trade enables better use of the world's economic resources than does national protectionism. Countries can concentrate on their respective strength and draw from their trade partners the goods they need, but do not produce. But there have always been objections against free trade.

The international trade system has always been encumbered by disparate accusations of unfair competition. The fear that foreign competitors use unfair methods, such as dumping, as and is widespread. If one were to believe all the charges of dumping that are made, then international trade would have been completely destroyed long ago. Great restraint should be exercised with respect to allegations of dumping if one is interested in maintaining an interweaving of international economic activities.

The Free Trade Oppsition Cloaks itself in Dumping Charges

The modern form of the struggle against free trade cloaks itself in the accusation of ecological dumping or social dumping. With this difficult subject matter, one should not make sweeping generalisations. These things also are not gone into in detail in what follows.

Environmental protection is an asset that every economy produces at the cost of other assets. The people's preferences for the asset of environmental protection probably varies from country to country. It is also completely legitimate and does not at all distort trade if the environmental provisions-in line with the different national preferences—vary from country to country.

In the rich western European economic region, one should guard against a new form of cultural imperialism. It is not for this part of the world to impose its preferences for environmental assets on other countries, especially Third World countries. Free world trade brings not only economic advantages. Even more important is its contribution to lasting world peace.

In view of world population growth, every standstill in the movement towards a peaceful world society must be seen as a step backwards. We are compelled to run a race between the growing problems and the development of stable institutions to overcome them peacefully at global level. Economic history since the end of the Second World War shows clearly that free trade under the old GATT was of decisive importance for the prosperity of the industrialised nations.

The principle of help for self-help has nowhere been applied so consistently as on the free world market. In reverse, the examples of countries that cut themselves off from the world market show the disastrous consequences of the rigidity of a society which shuns the pressure of international competition.

Revolutionary Success of Open-Market Policies

The West's policy of open markets pursued since 1948 and reinforced since 1989 has led to a dynamism which, in the true meaning of the word, is revolutionary. More than half the word population now lives in countries with annual

GDP growth rates of more than 5 per cent. Europe is not among that group, which may be why it also stands somewhat apart in its mentality.

Certainly, there also can be undesirable trends in free trade. There is not ideal systems; one must choose between imperfect potentialities. However, no realistically better substitute for the free trade system is in sight, not even with respect to the goals of a pacified world: an ecological sound world economy and a balance of global dimensions between the poor and the rich. An ideal government of philosopher kings armed with absolute power certainly could do some thing better than does free trade—but such a government remains fictitious. There are tangible and narrow limits to what the political system, whether democratic or not, can effect in a positive sense. This is how the structural conservatism of democratic and other political systems impedes the timely assertion of reforms necessary to achieve a world peace society.

The GATT was turned into the World Trade Organisation (WTO) a few years ago. Besides extending the free trade principle to services and additional agricultural sectors the new agreement foresees above all the full inclusion of the Third World in the system. The agreement commits the industrialised nations to open their markets to developing and threshold countries.

Other important points are the strengthening and tightening of the dispute mediation process. Based on a system of relatively independent ad hoc panels, it permits complaints against WTO member countries for violations of the agreement. Thus, what is arising here is an effective global jurisdiction within the meaning of a peaceful world domestic policy.

Exclusion as Penalty

The decisive sanction mechanism of the WTO—which is not a specialist organisation of the United nations—is the threat of exclusion. Exclusion would deny the penalised country free access to the markets of WTO members on the basis of most favoured nation status. This is a threat that requires no armed force, but is very effective. No country can still afford to do without the beneficial effects on prosperity that participation in international trade brings.

Thus, with the threat of denial of access to world markets for violating WTO rules, and the guarantee of a more or less fair competition for a country's own products for abiding by them, a non-military sanctions system has come into being. That is substantial progress on the path to a pacified world.

Certainly, this sanction system's sphere of influence is limited for the time being. Essentially, it will be used to assert the game rules of free trade. It offers no legal grounds for pressing other goals, such as on human rights. Attempting to expand it in this direction would for the foreseeable future put the entire system at risk.

In the current debate on globalisation, the question arises of whether the world economic institutions should not be converted in this manner, that politics regains its autonomy, and that the primacy of politics can be restored. The critics of globalisation point to the constraints to adjust which the world economy exercises on national or continental politics. However well this demand for the primacy of politics may be justified in philosophical terms, it virtually comes down to a demand for the ascendancy of the conservative principle.

Danger of a Slowed-Down World Integration

The demand for the primacy of politics is gaining strength from the desire to avoid the pressure to adjust which the dynamics of world events are exerting. It is today a conservative, and in fact a reactionary, longing for the (Utopian) return of the functioning European welfare state of two or three decades ago. If it were asserted, it would mean practically slowing down world integration. It would run dead against the goal of a world policy based on a desire for peace.

The present primacy of the economy over politics—in terms of the free movement of goods, services and capital—

is basically nothing more than the priority of the global principle over the provincial, the national principle. As such, it gives the principle of change pre-eminence over the principle of maintaining the status quo. What gives the primacy of the economy its legitimacy? Probably not the thought that world peace and better be secured by this means. Its legitimation lies in the very indirect economic success that the free trade system delivers. For the reflective observer, the question remains of whether this legitimation is sufficient.

To answer this question, however, and particularly if one pleads for maintaining the ascendancy of the economy, it appears appropriate to outline the consequences that can be expected from further integration of the world economy. As can be seen today in East and Southeast Asia, the growth dynamics of the world economy will lead to a marked rise in the living standards of a large part of the Third World.

Do Not Exclude Poor Countries from the Competition

The global consequences of Asia's growth should not have been seen only negatively. While it also may mean, for example, a great burden on the global climate, it leads at the same time to an acceleration of the process of falling birth rates and thus to an earlier stabilisation of the world population. Prosperity for the Third World is so far the only realistic answer to the urgent problem of population growth. And free competition on the world market in the only reliable means of achieving this prosperity in the course of some decades.

Despite ecological sacrifice in the medium term, continuation of Third World growth is the only way to solve the long-term ecological problems. One also should not forget that only those who can eat their fill and have a roof over their heads are prepared to reflect on ecology and discuss it.

As for the rest, the balance between rich and poor is more acceptable when the poor become richer than when the rich become poorer. That applies also at the international level. The market and access to it are peaceful sanctions of the world economic system on the basis of free trade. Those who are hungry and have nothing more to lose are more of a danger to world peace than those who have eaten their fill. The ruse of covering up domestic problems by cross border military aggression will become less attractive to the degree that a country's own economy is integrated in the global economic system. The more countries are economically dependent on each other, the more unlikely it is that they will wage war on each other.

Globalisation by free trade according to the principles of the WTO offers the only realistic opportunity to integrate the world peacefully and in time to prevent a major disaster. The primacy of the economy is the most important vehicle for a successful world domestic policy.

5

Export Subsidies:

A Distortion to Free Trade in Agriculture

Export subsidies are generally considered one of the most distorting trade tools used by governments to interfere with commerical markets. Export subsidies allow a government to determine the level and direction of trade solely on the basis of government subsidies, lowering world prices and denying sales for other, more competitive exporters. Not only are export subsidies unfair commercial tools, but, by encouraging surplus production, they encourage adverse environmental practices, waste government budgets, and may delay restructuring and reform of domestic industries. Substantial progress toward eliminating export subsidies will be a critical element of the World Trade Organisation (WTO) negotiations scheduled to begin at the end of this year.

The Situation Today

Under the Uruguay Round Agreement, countries agreed to strictly limit the use of export subsidies. First, products that had not benefited from export subsidies in the past were banned from receiving them in the future. Second, where countries had provided export subsidies in the past, their future use was capped and gradually reduced over 6 to 10 years. Developed countries were required to cut their spending on export subsidies by 36 per cent over six years while also reducing subsidised export quantities by at least 21 per cent on a commodity-specific basis.

Developing countries have until 2005 to cut spending by 24 per cent and subsidised quantities by 14 per cent. Third, countries agreed not to create new schemes that serve as disguised subsidies to get around the product-specific limits. Finally, countries recognised that export credit and food aid programmes were different and exempted them from the new budget and quantity limits, although there was agreement to negotiate disciplines on export credit programmes to ensure that they do not undermine WTO commitments.

Today, the European Union (EU) is the primary export subsidiser—accounting for nearly 85 per cent of the world total. Nearly all other countries agreed in the last round of negotiations not to use or to have only limited resource to use export subsidies. EU farmers, responding to domestic prices that are often twice the world price, produce more products than can be consumed in Europe, but at such high prices that they can be sold abroad only with generous subsidies. These subsidies force other competitors out of the market and discourage production in countries with comparative advantage.

If the EU's extravagant domestic subsidies are the root cause of export subsidies, they are also putting serious pressure on the whole EU system. The need to impose budgetary discipline on EU farm programmes (annual cost, about $46 billion) is becoming increasingly evident, even in Europe, and the EU's goal of epanding its membership to new countries is putting pressure on it to bring its farm programmes into line with other countries, which will help reduce its need to rely on export subsidies in the future.

Areas for Resolution

The upcoming negotiations should continue the work begun in the Urguay Round and eliminate existing export subsidies. There is no economic justification for their continued use. By removing subsidized exports, world prices should increase, and farmers, particularly in the EU, will not be artificially encouraged to overproduce products that they cannot grow competitively.

In addition to eliminating export subsidies, countries should examine the rules defining export subsidies to ensure that countries do not resort to other policy tools that might allow governments to distort markets. Specially, WTO members should to look closely at curbing agricultural state trading export monopolies that can exert undue market power or dispose of surplus commodities on a nonmarket basis. A recent WTO victory by the United States and New Zealand over Canada's special-class system of dairy exports shows that the existing rule against circumvention are effective but must be enforced.

Export credit and food aid programmes were addressed in the Uruguay Round agreement in recognition of the fact that those tools could be disguised as subsidies. These policies may again be on the agenda when the WTO negotiations commence next time. It will be important to ensure that the world's needy continue to have access to imported products, even when financial turmoil roils world markets and limits the ability of developing countries to meet their food and fibre needs.

Certain large exporting nations—primarily in the EU have used export taxes as a supply management tool by intervening in the market to restrict exports when domestic stocks are low. These measures can wreak havoc in international markets, exacerbating price swings and reducing the confidence of net-food-importing countries to abandon trade barriers and rely on the international market to provide food security. Similarly, some exporting countries use differential export taxes to discourage exports of basic products (such as grains or oilseeds); they force exporters to process the product domestically (into flour or oil and meal, for example) and export the value added products.

6

Add Value, Go Global:

Can Southern Firms Break into Export Markets?

The global economy has changed beyond recognition over the last decade. Widespread economic policy reform and in particular trade liberalisation have open up new opportunities for developing countries. In poor countries, however, the consequences of trade liberalisation are not always positive. What can the private sector do to respond better and make the most of new trading opportunities? What factors have limited the impact of economic reforms on export performance?

Why have exports from poorer countries failed to increase more rapidly following trade liberalisation? What can be done to improve performance? Research on the response of firms in the private sector to economic reform can underpin new approaches to export promotion for poorer developing countries. For a long time, protective trade policies, poorly performing state-owned industries and state controls over the private sector were blamed for poor export performance in Africa and South Asia. Now that some of these problems have been remedied, other obstacles have come to light.

The effect of economic liberalisation and adjustment on the performance of poor countries has been cause for concern. Trade liberalisation should increase incentives to export and facilitate business enterprise by encouraging private ownership through privatisation and by attracting foreign investment. Macroeconomic stability ought to boost business confidence and performance. All these factors should promote exports, offsetting job and income losses caused by the closure or reorganisation of inefficient enterprises and industries yet, although some degree of reform and stability it is without export growth that was expected.

Trade reform and macroeconomic stability may be necessary conditions for improved export performance put by them are insufficient. The obstacles to improving export performance are numerous and there is no easy policy answer. The research programme examined export performance at three levels.

- Regional: how trade strategies should vary with skills and natural resource endowments
- National: factors influencing the export performance of manufacturing
- Sectoral: the performance of particular sectors of the economy.

The East Asian economies have shown that developing countries can complete successfully in global markets. For many, they provide a blueprint for economic growth applicable to many poor countries

South Asia's comparative advantage lies in its abundant unskilled labour, while Africa's lies in its abundant natural resources. Different export promotion strategies are essential. South Asia's best prospectus are in labour-intensive manufacturing: the region's low level of exports would soar over the next decade if current obstacles to trade were reduced. Africa's exports could also increase but its biggest potential in primary products that need little educated labour and abundant natural resources.

Some African countries could also be substantial exporters of manufacturers, but their actual manufactured exports in most cases now fall far short. Comparing Ghana to Mauritius—one of Africa's most successful exporters of manufactured goods differences in firm-level efficiency are apparent Mauritian firms have more capital per worker and use it more efficiently. Reducing trade barriers is not sufficient. Wages in Ghana would have to be substantially lower to offset low labour productivity. Alternatively, labour productivity will have to be drastically improved if Ghanian firms are to compete successfully in export markets with wages at current levels.

Even when companies use capital and labour efficiently, poor infrastructure is a frequent stumbling products to export markets—an acute problem in landlocked countries and equally acute for manufacturers as research on Uganda clearly shows. What huts manufacturing exporters is being hit by the high cost of transporting their output to foreign markets and of transporting the materials they need from abroad. The cost penalties resulting from geography and poor infrastructure are far greater in Uganda than from high tariffs and other import restrictions.

Southern firms can still break into export markets, however, developing—country firms do export to markets with exacting standards for product quality, reliability of delivery, and consumer safety. Two crucial aspects, however, are often overlooked:

- Non-manufacturing sectors, such as tourism and horticulture, generate significant employment and offer opportunities for supplying increasingly sophisticated products. Although manufacturing is considered more attractive, certain areas of tourism and horticulture can be equally appealing.
- New export opportunities are created as southern producers establish closer links with foreign customers. Producers of labour-intensive products such as garments, horticulture and footwear frequently depend on large retailers and specialist international traders for designs, information about demand and technical support.

Supermarkets make key decisions about which fruits and vegetables to grow, how they should be produced and processed and which firms should be included in the business.

Strategic decisions by international producers and retailers in the footwear industry have been crucial in developing new production locations such as Vietnam and Romania. Similarly, work on automotive components production in South Africa and India illustrates how global sourcing by the leading motor companies closes off some markets and opens up others. Export prospects can only be evaluated in the light of global restructuring in these industries.

Emphasising global linkages does not mean that developing countries are powerless in the face of global forces. Even in tightly-structured industries, there is scope for national policy and national strategy. Further more, there are important export sectors that are not structured in this way. Some tourism is dominated by large northern firms and is heavily import-dependent, but there is also enormous potential and national policy will be crucial in shaping the industry and its contribution to the economy as a whole.

For southern firms to break into export markets, certain issues must be addressed, especially in Africa. Some are recognised as important policy issues—investing in human capital and improving infrastructure for example. As one set of constraints are reduced—such as removing policy—induced distortions through trade liberalisation—another set takes precedence. In response to the integration of global markets, southern producers must join the global distribution chains to ensure markets for their exports.

These findings impose hard choice on developing countries. Should a firm allocate limited funds for investment in human capital or investment infrastructure? Future research might contribute by quantifying relative rates of return. On another level, countries may worry about the independence and autonomy of local producers if they are to join a global chain typically donated by northern companies. Rules regulate governmental trade and investment policies but who controls the global buyers and multinatinal companies whose decisions have such huge impacts on developing countries?

7

World Trade Organisation

Affirming that "the establishment of the World Trade Organisation (WTO) ushers in a new era of global economic cooperation, reflecting the widespread desire to operate in a fairer and more open multilateral trading system for the benefit and welfare of their people," more than a hundred ministers in the ancient trading crossroads of Marrakesh signed the Final Act of the Uruguay Round and made decisions ensuring a running start for the WTO.

In the ornate Salle Royal of the Palaisdes Congress, the ministers, one by one, signed. The Final Act containing 28 agreements and appended to by some 26,000 pages of national tariff and services schedules, which GATT economists estimate will add some US $ 755 billion to world exports and raise incomes by some $ 235 billion annually.

Several ministers also signed the new Government Procurement Code that was negotiated in parallel with the Uruguay Round and three other plurilateral agreements: on dairy products, bovine meat and civil aircraft. The ceremony effectively marked the start of the transition from GATT to the WTO.

In the Marrakesh Declaration they had adopted just hours earlier, the Ministers had saluted as "a historic achievement" the conclusion of the round, which strengthen the world economy, lead to more trade, investment, employment and income growth throughout the world". They had also expressed their determination to "resist protectionist pressures of all kinds". In this regard, they pledged, with immediate effect and until the establishment of the WTO, not to "take any trade measures that would undermine or adversely affect the results of the Uruguay Round negotiation or their implementation."

Ministerial Decisions

The establishment of a Preparatory Committee for the WTO was one of the four decisions taken by ministers. The other three were: the Decision on Acceptance of the Accession to the Agreement Establishing the World Trade Organisation; the Decision on Trade and Environment; and the Decision on Organisational and Financial Consequences flowing from Implementation of the Agreement Establishing the WTO.

The Preparatory Committee, to be headed by Mr. Peter Sutherland in his personal capacity, will be in charge of ensuring an orderly transition from the GATT to the WTO. Its remit is to ensure the efficient operation of the WTO immediately as of the date of its establishment. Thus, it will convene and prepare the Implementation Conference, which will decide formally on the date of entry into force of the WTO Agreement.

Opening Ceremonies

"Our meeting here in Marrakesh takes place at the close of the most ambitious trade negotiations in world economic history - we should be proud of this stride towards a more open world which will be, through the dynamism of exchanges between nations and the lifting of barriers and protectionist regulations, a source of prosperity and welfare for the people worldwide," said His Royal Highness the Crown Prince Sidi Mohammed at the opening of the Ministerial Meeting. He stressed that "we all are witnessing here in Marrakesh what will be the legal and institutional pillar of international Trade in the twenty–first century."

The TNC Chairman at Ministerial level, Minister Sergio Abreau Bonilla (Uruguay), opened the Ministerial Meeting by reminding participants that the real effectiveness of the new trade rules depended on the political will of governments. "We must therefore strengthen our determination to honour the commitments which we will assume with the signature of the Final Act," he said. Minister Abreau added: "Behind each signature, there are millions of workers, farmers, industrialists, professionals and businessmen who harbour the hope that the results of the Round will create new horizons for trade, employment and investment and offer better possibilities of tackling poverty and recession, the paving the way for the economic and social development of nations."

Sutherland's Report

"Few trading caravans can have viewed this beautiful city with as much pleasure and as much relief—as ours does. But then very few trading caravans were on the road for more than seven years, and none carried such a priceless cargo. This week you as Ministers will sign the greatest trade agreement in history, one whose benefits span entire continents and a wide range of trade sectors alike," the TNC Chairman at Officials Level, GATT Director—General Peter Sutherland said.

Mr. Sutherland reported that the work of the TNC since the successful conclusion of the Uruguay Round negotiations on 15 December 1993 had been focused on the preparations for the Marrakesh Meeting. First, the Final Act Embodying the Results of the Uruguay Round of Multilateral Trade Negotiations was legally rectified, agreed and circulated to all participants. Secondly, the schedules of market access commitments in goods and services and the MFN exemption lists in services were multilaterally verified for attachment to the Marrakesh Protocol. Thus the Final Act, rectified and completed by the verified schedules, was now well as trade and investment.

Reflecting on the successful conclusion of the negations, US Trade Representative Michael Kantor said he was "struck by the thin line that separates success and failure... (but) we succeeded because the ties that bind us together are strong than the forces seeking to pull us apart." He stressed that "our vision of the trading system must be dynamic and able to meet the emerging challenges to our collective global economic growth." Thus, "increasingly, we will address issues related to each other's internal policies, such as competition policy and other domestic regulatory policies, as well as environmental protection and labour standards."

Canada's Trade Minister, Mr. Roy MacLaren, emphasised that when WTO is asked to tackle new trade policy issues, it should proceed in a manner consistent with its competence and mandate. He warned that "when examining new issues, we must, for example be wary of being seduced by the argument that differing approaches to issues such as environmental protection constitute an unfair train practice justifying some form of action—new issues can become a vehicle for new protectionism." Minister MacLaren stressed that "to fall victim in the World Trade Organisation to the narrow interest groups who favour trade sanctions as the instrument of choice to force nations to comply with the policies of other would be to abandon some of the most fundamental gains we have made."

Development Goals

India's Minister of Commerce, Mr. Pranab Mukherjee, warned that the acute differences between levels of development and incomes among nations have "enough latent heat to melt down the most elaborately engineered structures." Thus, "the long-term survival of the multilateral trading system will depend upon reducing the present inequities." Regarding new issues, Minister Mukherjee said while India was strongly committed to internationally—recognised labour standards, it could not see any merit in linking this subject to international trade. On the other hand, he attached importance to an examination in the Preparatory Committee of the relationship between immigration policies and international trade.

Bangladesh' Minister for Commerce, Mr. M. Shamsul Islam, speaking on behalf of the least-developed countries, hoped that "in the implementation of the Uruguay Round Agreements, the international community will be more responsive to the needs of the most disadvantaged group of nations." He urged a comprehensive assessment of the

Uruguay Round results with "any imbalances ... to be redressed through appropriate action including additional trade preferences, development assistance and debt relief." Minister Islam pointed to the "need by LLDCS for substantial technical assistance in the implementation of the results of the Round. On new issues, he supported the consideration of the relationship between movements of natural persons and international trade in the Preparatory Committee.

Zimbabwe"s Minister of Industry and Commerce, Dr. H. Murerwa, said that his country's preliminary evaluation of the Uruguay Round results suggested gains for certain products, stand–still position for others and potential losses for some products as a result of erosion of EC trade preferences. However, he believed that "the process of liberalisation will in the long–run strengthen the global trading system and benefit the peoples of both the developed and developing countries." Minister Murerwa said the challenge fracing the developing countries is "to expand and diversify our export capabilities as well as strengthening the international competitiveness of our products." Reready for signature by Ministers. Simultaneously, the TNC at official level had approved for adoption by Ministers four Decisions and Marrakesh Declaration.

The GATT Director-General said that "the signature ceremony will be a just cause for celebration not only because its represents signing—off on the Uruguay Round, but because it will be signing—on to the work of putting the results into effect and ensuring that their potential is used to the fullest."

Early Ratification Urged

Many Ministers underlined the urgency of ratifying the Uruguay Round agreements to enable the World Trade Organisation to be fully operational.

EC Commissioner Sir Leon Brittan emphasised that: "each of us, by our signature at Marrakesh, pledges himself or herself to submit the results of the Uruguay Round for formal approval in accordance with our domestic laws and, equally important, to proceed without delay to implement in our domestic laws, the commitments we made during the negotiations" He said one proof of the quality of those commitments was "the ever—lengthening queue of candidates for accession to the GATT and to the WTO." The EC Commissioner suggested that the WTO tackle the following issues: ensuring intensive cooperation between the WTO and the IMF and the World Bank; addressing urgently the interface between trade and the environment; working with the International Labour Office and other organisations, the WTO must address problems such as child exploitation, forced labour or the denial to workers of free speech or free association; and distortion of trade which can be caused by different standards of competition law and practice in different countries.

Japan's Deputy Prime Minister and Minister for Foreign Affairs Mr. Tsutomu Hata, underlined the importance of the Round's conclusion "in securing confidence in the world economic order." He recalled that his country had made significant contributions to the Round, including acceptance of the Agreement on Agriculture and cutting average tariffs on industrial and mining products by 61 per cent to rate as low as 1.5 per cent. "As a result of the Uruguay Round, the Japanese market offers greater opportunities for success by foreign exporters depending upon their efforts," he added. Minister Hata expressed strong support for the early entry into force of the WTO Agreement, and suggested that the WTO consider additional issues closely related to trade, including regionalism as grading the WTO, he viewed "Marrakesh as the stating platform which will put in place a strong rule–based multilateral trading system that should safeguard the interest of all nations, weak and strong."

The Swiss Minister of Public Economy, Mr. J. P. Delamuraz, pointed out that "by concluding the Uruguay Round, we have taken a decisive step towards the adaptation of the multilateral trading system to contemporary economic realities." This had meant for many participant "substantial adjustments" in domestic economic policy, and for Switzerland reforms in its agricultural policy. "We have added a number of stones to the foundations of a system of multilateral management of the world economy," said Mr. Delamuraz, "we have also recognise the interdependence that is binding us ever more closely together." He noted with special satisfaction the confirmation in the Marrakesh Declaration of the "need for positive measures on behalf of the developing countries, and especially of the least developed among them, as well as the desirability of possible additional measures for their benefit." Mexico's Secretary for Trade and Industrial Development, Mr. Jaime Serra Puche, lauded the result of the Round as signifying "recognition" of the adjustment measures that have been taken up by many developing countries to open their economies. He believed that the results "will further the creation of new jobs and growth in the wage levels of our workers." Secretary Puche stressed that "protection of the environment and workers' rights must go hand in hand with efforts to liberalise world trade, for progress in liberalisation to improve the environment and the well-being of workers," but warned against these subject being used as pretexts for "desguised trade protectionism."

Brazil's Minister of External Relations, Mr. Celso Amorium, said that the Uruguay Round "will be remembered as the first one in which developing countries had an active participation in the course of the whole negotiating process." he underlined that "We, the developing countries, have bet on trade liberalisation and on the multilateral trading system ... Even though our organisation does not bear the word development in its name, it will lose much of its purpose if its rules and disciplines do not contribute to freeing hundreds of millions of human beings from poverty and misery."

The Czech Republic's Minister of Industry and Trade, Mr. Vladimir Dlouhy, highlighted the importance his country attached to "the full integration of the economies in transition into the multilateral trading system." Pointing to these countries' need for better access to markets and fair application of trade and competition rules, he urged that the "the role of the multiateral trading system in this process should be made more effective and more visible."

Singapore's Minister for Trade and Industry, Mr. Yeo Cheow Tong, said "the signing of the Final Act does not mean the end... the challenge now is to see through the successful establishment of the WTO and the implementation of the agreement." Minister Yeo said that Singapore fully supported the WTO because it "has long recognised that the free market system is way to economic growth and prosperity for our people." In line with this, he extended his country's invitation to host the first Ministerial Meeting of the WTO. "This will be the first time a major global trade meeting will be held in Asia, and will complete the circle of Uruguay Round meetings that began in South America in Uruguay, then moved on the North America, to Europe and today in Marrakesh, Africa," he added.

Conclusion

At the conclusion of the Ministerial Meeting Minister Abreau noted that many of the one hundred ministers who have spoken had stressed that "notwithstanding the tumultuous economic and political events of the past seven – and – a – half years, all participants have undertaken considerable efforts to improve conditions of market access." Noteworthy too had been "the engagement of the developing and least-developed countries in the process of countributing their share to the global effort to reduce trade barriers."

Another major theme was "the role that multilateral cooperation must play as the foundation for trade relations amongst nations." Min. Abreau said that to implement this principle on a permanent basis, "all had agreed that the results of the negotiations constituted a single undertaking, based on the WTO as a new international institution." He added that one decision taken at the meeting was the convening of an Implementation Conference later in the year.

In the course of the meeting, the TNC Chairman said ministries had stressed the importance they attached to the examination in the Preparatory Committee of the following subjects for inclusion in the WTO agenda: the relationship between the trading system and internationally recognised labour standards; the relationship between immigration policies and international trade; trade and competition policy, including rules on export financing and restrictive business practices; trade and investment; regionalism; the interaction between trade policies and policies relating to financial and monetary matters, including debt and commodity markets; international trade and company law; the establishment of a mechanism for compensation for the erosion of preferences; the link between trade, development, political stability and the alleviation of poverty; and unilateral or extraterritorial trade measures.

8

The Dematerialisation of the World Economy

The first Industrial Revolution marked the transition from robber – and – plunder colonialism to the systematic development of the "overseas" territories in the framework of the international division of labour between raw materials suppliers and manufacturers of finished goods. There was an "historic integration" of the colonised areas in the development of their parent—states. What will the third Industrial Revolution do for the Third World ? Will it now come to an "historic separation" ?

The end of the East-West conflict was reason enough to talk about a radical change in world politics. But at the same time an upheaval in the world economy is taking place that possibly will have even wider impacts. As a reference point for the following thoughts, three dimensions of this change are pointed out:

1 The upgrading of processing information rather than materials as object of economic activity (technological dimension) ;

2 the evolvement of global communications networks (sociocultural dimension) ;

3 the change of the nature of work (socio-economic dimension).

All three dimensions can be summarised under the buzzphrase "tertialisation of the world economy."

In that respect, talk of the "Third Industrial Revolution" is misleading. It is not about a third epoch of industrialisation, but about the beginning of a de–industrialisation, the transition from the industrial to the information society.

Historic Separation?

In the 1960s and early 1970s, there was often talk of the Third World as the Third Sector of the world economy. Also then the Third World was not much more than an "imaginary community". But as such it had a certain significance in world politics. This implied not only its strategic role in the East-West conflict and its ideological function as the supporter of different "third paths" between capitalism and socialism. It was also about the Third World's attested "chaos power". That linked the fear (in the North) and the hope (in the South) that the developing countries would be in a position to cut off the industrial nations from supplies of important raw materials, thus putting them under pressure. But it was soon seen that both sides had over estimated this possibility, even with regard to oil. Instead of supply bottlenecks arising, raw materials prices plummeted. For some commodities, the fall in prices exceeded those of the Great Depression of 1929/30.

This was due, inter alia, to the conjunction of lower demand from the industrial nations and expansion of production by the raw materials suppliers. Business activities dependent upon the supply of raw materials are tending to lose importance compared with the overall development of the global economy. The reason for this is to be seen in the transition from a material to an information economy.

This transition is taking place in line with the revolutionizing of data transmission and the expansion of financial transactions which are not directly related to changes in the production of materials. The speed of the changes is remarkable.

However, the dematerialisation of business activities does not lead to decoupling of the Third World from the world economy. Declining market shares in world trade are not the expression of separation, but a loss of the affected countries positions in the world economy. Thus, the impact of dematerialisation is "only" that the negotiating positions of raw materials suppliers vis–a–vis the industrial nations will deteriorate further.

Differentiation of the Third World

But the radical change in the global economy is affecting some developing countries worse than others. Sub–saharan Africa, and some countries in West and South Asia and Latin America are being pushed back further. The oil–producing countries with their high per capita export earnings will be able to hold their positions in the world economy for some time to come. The threshold countries of East and South-East Asia can expand theirs so long as they can continue to attract a growing share of global industrial production, and at the same time participate in the tertialisation of the world economy in the shape of rapidly-growing financial transactions. Thereby it should be noted that the degree of tertialisation in itself is not an adequate indicator for economic avant-gardism. Brazil exhibits a high degree of tertialisation in combination with a low macroeconomic development dynamics. A good part of its tertialisation is being achieved by speculative financial transactions with their inherently greater risks and uncertainties than in the industrial countries. Such dangers have been demonstrated by Mexico's peso crisis and its repercussions on the whole of Latin America.

In some Third World countries, a "location annuity" has replaced the old raw materials one. Here it's about providing locations for off-shore transactions which offer international capital traders a maximum of freedom of movement combined with low taxation. Suitable for such operations are small countries which, despite low levy rates, achieve significant income in macroeconomic terms.

The radical changes in the world economy are spurring the differentiation of the Third World Without, however, necessarily fostering a dissolution of the Third World as an "imaginary community". It is precisely the advanced countries of East and South-East Asia that are showing a certain interest in the formulation of joint positions of the "South" in order to secure their own positional gains in the global economy. It's not by chance that the non-aligned countries and the Group of 77 have formed a joint coordination committee, and that the ASEAN countries are changing course on the international human rights policy.

Hitherto, the developing countries' strategy was to broaden the concept of human rights as a justification for demands on the industrial nations. But of late some developing countries, led by the ASEAN states, have questioned the universal validity of human rights even after their universality was confirmed by consensus at the Conference on Human Rights in Vienna in 1993. Playing a role in this policy is the governments' fear that due to the expansion of global communications networks, the behaviour patterns and preferences of their own people could in some way become similar to those of the West. As the rulers see it, that would be detrimental to the continuation of the development models practised so far.

Internet Creates New Cultural Dimension

Much information which Asian governments view as subversive in already globally available on the Internet. The old struggle over the world information order, which at first was primarily a clinch between East and West, is thus taking on a new dimension. For with the growing importance of computer literacy to a country's ability to assert itself on world markets, the Asian threshold countries have not only an interest in controlling the on-line communication but also to expand it and the know-how that it requires.

Even the critics of any interventions in the internet and other global communications networks must admit that modern communications technologies are politically blind and their use in itself does not represent progress. The setting up and expansion of global information highways will offer forum not only to people who want to use it for education and enlightenment, but also to all shades of fundamentalists. These highways will not necessarily bring the misery of many Third World regions closer to the industrial countries, but possibly rather strengthen the tendency to process all world events as entertainment.

Global Two-thirds Society

The gravest aspect of the current upheaval in the world economy is its negative impact on jobs. The information economy needs for fewer workers than an economy based on materials. Instead, the demands on the skills of the workers are growing. Twenty per cent of the world workforce will in future be employed as (overworked) "intelligence workers". Eighty per cent will work part–time, if they are not underemployed or jobless. So the tertialisation of the global economy delivers more underemployment rather than more leisure time. The workers who are rationalised out of their jobs in the industrial sector cannot be absorbed by the service sector because it, too, is not left untouched by rationalisation measures. The civil service is also cutting back on staff. At all levels, there's a race to make the greatest possible savings on payrolls. At the same time, there's growing pressure to cut costs in providing for the victims of this development. That means thinning out the social security safety net.

The bottom line is that the two-thirds society, which developmental action groups hitherto assumed was limited to the Third World, is spreading worldwide. That, however, will not in the foreseeable future lead to an amendment of the North-South disparities. It's true that the change in the global economy is taking place faster, and to a greater extent in the industrial nations. But rationalisation is also happening in the developing countries in a bid to boost their competitiveness. So the upheaval in the world economy aggravates the problems which exist in a majority of the developing countries, while creating new ones in the industrial nations. The need for action on the North-South policy is growing, while the industrial nations. The need for action on the North-South Policy is growing, while the industrial nations' scope for concessions and compromises is shrinking. The new social question which is now crystallizing at global level is not being answered. The consequences are unforeseeable.

Another Loser?

It's more probable that a sharpening of the North–South confrontation is to be reckoned with. For the industrial nations will attempt to keep the social costs of the information economy at bay for as long as possible. The trade unions will thereby compete with the developing countries for jobs for their members. But this policy has its limits precisely because of the peaking of the problems in the industrial nations. Overstepping these limits means war, and passively accepting them chaos and social decay. Solutions could be sought in two directions: effective taxation of the information economies, and the creation of jobs in the non-profit sector. But it's possible there are no global solutions for global problems. That would mean for at least part of the Third World a renewal of the old debate on partial decoupling from the world economy.

9

The Role of Financial Markets and the IMF:

The Genesis of Asia's Financial Crisis

It is obvious that the major causes of Asia's financial crisis were rooted in the affected countries. The evils were excessive foreign borrowing, poor supervision of banks, and overvaluation of national currencies. Apart from those policy failures, however, there were external factors. These were, besides the instability of the international finance markets, above all the wrong reaction of the International Monetary Fund, which aggravated the crisis rather than counteracting it. The role of the IMF must be fundamentally redefined.

The Asian crisis marks for the time being the end of the Southeast and East Asian economic miracle of the last four decades. Engulfed by the malaise of the worst—hit countries, Thailand, Indonesia and South Korea, the entire region in suffering economic weakness and in part even a decline in economic performance. The question is whether the Asian crisis could have been avoided or whether wrong economic policy decisions gave it a kick—start.

The Causes of the Crisis

Analysis of the causes for the Asian crisis have to date been marked by an astonishing one—sidedness. Up front, explanations emphasise the internal causes, particularly the private sector's excessive foreign borrowing. But two other factors played central, if not decisive, roles in the spread of the crisis. One was the great Volatility of the international capital markets, the other the inappropriate policies of the IMF.

This article analysis these three major causes of the crisis. Another question is how in future one can prevent manageable economic problems getting out of hand and developing into a crisis that threatens more than the economic stability of single countries.

But a closer look shows that the crisis, which broke out in mid—1997, has assumed such an unforeseen dimension that individual corrective measures of economic policy can no longer cope with it. A huge structural economic crisis has arisen. What developments led to it ?

Foreign Borrowing

Let us look first at the high private sector borrowing abroad. With hindsight, it is easy to pass judgement on it as having been wrong and dangerous. But that does not mean that private foreign borrowing is harmful in general. If it finances profitable investments, it is merely the use of foreign savings when domestic savings are too low. IMF reports also reflected this assessment.

We know from experience of earlier debt crisis that a high foreign indebtedness by the private sector is latently, but not generally, risky. The Asian crisis also has reconfirmed that international finance markets differentiate between individual private debtors and the credit—worthiness of national economies only in the case of a few countries. In smaller countries, including OECD member South Korea, difficulties in servicing individual loans lead to investors getting out of these markets. This is the real danger of large-scale private foreign debts.

That makes foreign loans much more expensive than domestic credits. If the national interest rate is higher than that of international market, cash deposit requirement often can be an adequate incentive to borrow at home or take out a longer-term loan. Both alternatives lead to greater stability of the domestic finance system, as the risk of withdrawal of capital at short notice, as in the case of the Asian crisis countries, is much reduced.

Instability of the Finance Markets

Beyond the cash deposit requirement, however, further restructuring must be done in the finance sectors of the Asian crisis economies and threshold and developing countries. Frequently, they are demands for greater transparency. Improved banking supervision and, especially in the case of South Korea, a broader diversification of shareholding. These steps are important, but they will not prevent the next crisis because they do not put an end to the instability of the international finance markets.

The Asian crisis has also reconfirmed that highly mobile capital can produce instability. It must seem dubious when there are calls (particularly by the IMF and US politicians involved in financial matters) for the pushing through of even more capital mobility as a consequence of the crisis. But even liberal economists are now increasingly questioning the ideal of a world without restrictions on the free movement of capital linked with an enhanced IMF mandate.

IMF Intervention

The IMF's policy intensified the volatility of the international capital flows, that is, their wide fluctuation margin. When American and European fund managers began to pull their capital out of Asia's crisis countries, Asian debtors fell into arrears in servicing their liabilities, and the currencies came under heavy pressure, the IMF ordered a drastic cure. This was aimed at lowering inflation rates and reducing government budget deficits. But as there were not critical inflaction rates, and government budgets were in fact, in surplus, this policy was more than odd. A quick look at the economic development in the Asian crisis countries illustrates the relatively positive situation of the three economies before the crisis broke out.

What Measures to Stabilise Currencies?

The IMF policy also manifrests deficiencies beyond the

measures it ordered. I shall not discuss here the question of whether it is wise and appropriate for the IMF to clamp measures and restrictions of private sector debtors and their governments while the creditors side can emerge from the crisis largely without loss.

But one must ask whether the IMF's measures to stabilise the currencies were suitable in an acute—crisis. They are mainly measures with individual impacts, giving priority to increasing real interest rates. The aim is to regain the trust of international finance markets and stimulate fresh loan flows to these countries. The long-term objective is to restore currency stability.

This policy, however, has to weaknesses. On the one hand, it sets indebted companies under more pressure as they must not only pay more for their foreign currency loans due to devaluation, but are also faced with higher domestic interest. On the other hand, while it is true that a high interest rate policy in countries with stable economies can have a positive impact in attracting capital, that is not so in countries suffering from an acute economic crisis, as Indonesia shows. Recovery of the exchange rate to a realistic level that would enable the companies to service their debts has not happened there.

The Future of the IMF

Having reflected upon the dubious results of the IMF policy, one is bound to ask what role the organisation should play in future. Should its task be to have a stabilising effect in a crisis, or should the IMF be an instrument to assert certain economic policy concepts?

The IMF itself has defined its current function very one—sidedly, focusing on its services for the international finance markets. According to a self-assessment in a internal IMF document, it sees itself performing a dual function as a 'confidental economic adviser' and as the 'watchdog for the international financial markets'. But the IMF does not by a long way give the attention they deserve to the interests of the 350 million people in the countries under its wing.

Criticism in the West

Criticism of the IMF is growing not only in the Asian crisis countries but also especially in the USA and more and more in Europe. Conservative American politicians such as the former US Secretary of State Charles Shultz have described the IMF as ineffective, unnecessary and obsolute. They have also proposed that the IMF be abolished at some time after the Asian crisis has been overcome. The IMF's current policy is also coming in for heavy criticism in the academic debate on the crisis, which is demanding a redefinition of the organisation's mandate.

Other possibilities are conceivable beyond the radical option of abolishing or privatising the IMF. The IMF should in any case be required to tackle the specific situations in the crisis countries with greater awareness of the affected countries. In the course of the Asian crisis, the option of creating a regional fund was also discussed, but the Western G7 countries and the IMF emphatically rejected it. One should, however, consider whether regional institutions could not in fact work more efficiently than an authority based in Washington with competence for the entire world.

A regional structure with several monetary funds could facilitate the overcoming of crisis situations, although only if a global structure were to be maintained alongside the regional components. This global body, a kind of world monetary council, would be composed of representatives of the US and European central banks and the regional funds. Besides taking over the IMF's current tasks, such an international regime could also deal with stabilising exchange rates between the industrialised nations and in particular with the development of a target zones system between the dollar and the Euro. The winners in a less unstable international finance system would be the developing and threshold countries that at present still need to take the questionable medicine prescribed by the IMF.

10

Development: *The People Know Best*

Meetings of the World Bank and the World Trade Organisation has inspired high—mined protest and, on occasion, even vandalism. But this protest and vandalism may miss the point. It is hard to blame those who complain of bullying or blundering by the great institutions of global power. But the poor of the world, especially the poor of developing countries, deserve more than street demonstrations. The poor understand better than anybody the complicated details of their own poverty – the absence of health care, the lack of education, and all the sinister perils to their own safety and well-being. They know the failures of their governments, and of international institutions.

And that is the point: It is the people of the poor countries who will have to apply new knowledge to design and achieve their own development. A country can only develop when its citizens have the freedom to address their own development problems. The obligation of the rich countries, is to give help where they can. And anyone who doesn't see a moral imperative to contribute to a fairer, more prosperous future is free to frame the obligation differently—as self—interest, for example. It will surely serve us better to invest in a peaceful and contented global community than to invite the strife and poverty of unanswered injustice and economic ruin.

Among our relevant conclusions: Powerful institutions of global finance and trade (not least, the World Bank and the World Trade Organisation) can be a source of real promise to poor countries. If governed right, they can help integrate developing economies into the enriching opportunities of global trade and investment. But such promise is often wasted because the very poverty of poor–country governments weakens their ability to negotiate the terms that would serve them best.

Communities in poor countries find themselves at a special disadvantage when it comes to bargaining with foreign investors. Investment can bring growth and spread wealth. It can also threaten human rights and social cohesion, or cultural integrity, and the fragile balance of ecosystems. Nobel economist Amartyasen has spoken powerfully about the intimate relation between development and choice, the subject of his thought—provoking book Development as Freedom. Development, Sen argues, "consists of the removal of various types of unfreedoms that leave people with little choice and little opportunity ..." He defines freedom as "both the primary end and the principal means of development."

A precondition of this freedom is knowledge—knowledge of the hard facts and the hard science on which real choices are constructed, Also it is knowledge of good governance—procedures of choice that are effective, responsive and democratic. For budgetary reasons, rich countries contribution in international development was severely cut in the 1990s. Now, along with others in the rich countries, they have to begin to reinvest in international development.

This means a new commitment to the improvement of lives, and to the future that the North must share with the South. It will be a reinvestment in peace, and in our own prosperity. This remains a matter of obligation, and of sensible self-interest.

11

Venture Capital For Small and Medium Business:

A Proposal for South-South Cooperation

Although great strides have been made in the last decade to help finance business start-ups for micro-enterprises in low-income countries (LICs), using models such as the Grameen Bank in Bangladesh and others, no similar initiative has been taken to help small and medium enterprises (SMEs) in these countries.

Development banks or other development finance institutions (DFIs) in developing countries are not really meant nor organised to serve the particular needs of their counties' SMEs. They are not only unable to draw on a local capital market to finance their operations, but they also lack the range of advisory services required by SMEs to submit bankable loan applications and are themselves ill-equipped to evaluate such applications. Consequently, they concentrate on a few large projects—preferably of the infrastructure type—for which they rely on the technical expertise of the foreign donors financing them or specially hired consultants.

In the absence of a realistic access to DFIs, SMEs have been constrained to seek their loans for new business ventures from commercial banks. The fact that since 1978 the World Bank has been challenging a large portion of its credit lines intended for SMEs through commercial banks rather than through DFIs, reflects the importance which donors attach to the role of LIC commercial banks as the principal intermediaries for SME lending.

Reasons for Failure of Traditional Banking Systems

However, there are several important reasons why commercial banks are ill-suited to perform this task. First and foremost, the banking systems of these countries were conceived during a period when most investment capital was provided by the government, usually drawing on foreign aid. Thus, even in those LICs which had not entirely succumbed to the socialist ideology in the sense of eliminating all private enterprise, commercial banks continue to limit their credit activity largely to self-liquidating, low-risk credits seldom exceeding 12 months's duration, preferably conventional trade credits. Secondly, even in the exceptional cases where commercial banks in these countries entertain applications for medium-term credits to finance the launching of a small manufacturing project, they will normally demand ironclad collateral in the forms of liens on real-estate and/or personal guarantees by friends and relatives with similar backing, unless the applicant is a well-known customer of the bank

Thirdly, with their overriding concern for profitability, most LIC commercial banks tend to like upon business start-up loans to SMEs as being too risky and/or administratively too costly to handle in relation to the loan amounts involved. For these reasons, commercial banks in these countries are unlikely to establish in-house facilities to meet the specific needs of SMEs, such as helping them in project preparation and market analysis. Last but not least, factors such as the project's development orientation" (e.g. its important substitution and export potential, its ability to increase productivity and its employment generation features) do not enter into the calculations of commercial banks which will orient their actions towards "bottom line" results and risk minimisation. Under the circumstances, most commercial banks are not inclined to become directly involved in project supervision, as long as their customer's repayment records are satisfactory.

Credit for SMEs

Whereas new approaches have been developed over the last decade by various development assistance agencies to help up-grade commercial banks' staff capability, especially in advising SME borrowers in such matters as project formulation and market analysis as well as improving their loan repayment capacity, only recently has an effort been made to find ways and means of making investment capital available to SME entrepreneurs for launching new businesses. In some LICs, lines of credit have been established by multilateral or bilateral banks from which loan capital can be sought for such projects, but only seldom has genuine risk (i.e., equity) capital been made available and when some only through the donors' own agencies. The interest rate charged by the local banks for administering loans from these credit lines in local currency are generally at par with existing commercial rates, which tend to be prohibitive for a new venture of the type being promoted. These high rates are due to several factors, including (a) the local rates of inflation and the consequent devaluation risks, (b) the high risk factor of the new enterprises with little or no collateral and credit standing, and (c) the lack of experience of bank staff in the evaluation of loan requests submitted to them for unfamiliar projects.Significantly, most international DFIs are loath to lower interest rates to be applied on loans financed by their credit lines, lest they be accused of unfair competition on the local financial markets.

Incentives Ineffective in Attracting Foreign Investors

Although many international conferences, investment promotion meetings and other fora have been staged by UN bodies and donor groups to generate private investor interest in the LICs, these efforts have proved largely ineffectual. While much has been done by LIC governments in recent years to create a more attractive "enabling environment" for private investment, these incentives have been necessary but not sufficient to convince developed—country enterprises or investors to assume the necessary risks, with the exception of selected sectors such as mineral extraction, tourism and a narrow range of exportable consumer goods, such as out-of-season fruits and vegetables, and tropical products such as cocoa and certain spices. Even public support for project preparation has ultimately failed to provide preparation private business in industrial countries the incentives needed to take an active role in a broadly-based economic development of LICs.

The bottom line for potential investors in LICs is constituted by the profits which their investment will yield within a reasonable period of time, under conditions which offer a reasonable amount of political and legal stability. So far, these basic conditions have not been met on the whole. In the new global economy with its almost total reliance on free market principles and the ability to choose investment sites freely, the choice is not likely to fall on the LICs, but rather on a small number of more advanced developing countries, apart from the industrial countries themselves.

South-to-South Technological/Commercial Cooperation

While the inherent disadvantages faced by LICs in competing for foreign investment capital are too great to be overcome by a magic panacea, any attempt at a solution must include measures designed to mobilise the entrepreneurial abilities and dynamism available in existing and potential SMEs engaged in production of a variety of goods destined for the broad consumer market at home and abroad. In most LICs such existing or potential SMEs need to access affordable foreign technologies, i.e., the machinery and the technological know-how required to install and make the machinery function. One of the prime sources of such technologies for LICs can be found in enterprises in South/Southeast Asia and China, countries that have only recently graduated from the LIC status (or have not yet done so but have nevertheless managed to create a modern industrial sector within their overall state of underdevelopment and poverty). The concretisation of transfers of technology from these countries to the LICs is especially affected by the financing problems described above, because in the normal case neither one of the potential partners can afford the necessary venture, even though they can and will invest their know-how, time and very often land, buildings and infrastructure. This problem is much less acute in the case of the more expensive, and hence often unaffordable "Northern" technologies, where the technology provider finds it easier to mobilise start-up capital from its won resources or by borrowing from his commercial bank against his firms' overall credit line.

The underlying economic rationale in favour of such South-to South, company-to company transfers of production technology argues that Asian firms can help launch industrial start-ups in these countries far more cheaply and quickly than the more sophisticated companies from the North. By offering labour-intensive rather than capital-intensive production machinery accompanied by vitally needed on the-job training, back-up managerial and maintenance follow-up at a fraction of the cost of Northern firms, Asian companies' Cooperation can spell the difference between a successful business start-up and a failed one. Furthermore Asian-sourced machinery can be operated at production scales corresponding to the reduced market requirements and limited purchasing power of most LIC markets.

In view of the above described financing problems faced by South-to-South deals, it is proposed that a Venture Capital Fund be established specializing in the provision of equity capital for joint ventures (JVs) among SMEs in various LICs. In many cases the existence of such a FUND—Which might be called the Venture Capital Fund or simply (VENCAP)—will spell the difference between business proposals that are still-born for want of the required initial financing, and profitable ventures which are launched thanks to the missing—if minority—equity contribution from the fund.

Characteristics of the FUND

The proposed VENCAP would be expected to be an active participant in the project in which it will invest, sharing its financial and strategic vision with the invested firm. To this end, it must have access to experienced project evaluation specialists with intimate knowledge of conditions in low-income countries in general, and the project and its promoters in particular. As might be expected, the FUND would concentrate its resources in early-state financing, rather than in plant expansion or replacement, inasmuch as the projects likely to be the most profitable are the new ones which will normally start from empty factory buildings and offices, where only a minimum amount of production equipment if any, is normally usable for the operation of the new JV.

The FUND would limit its participation to joint ventures in which firms of at least two developing countries hold equity stakes, although firms from developed countries might also participate. The FUND would limit its participation to production JVs whose total initial capital would not exceed a given sum to be determined. Its own participation would in turm also be limited by a relative ceiling per venture i.e., a maximum percentage of the total capital. This combination would implicitly set an absolute ceiling to the FUND's participation in any given JV.

Success and Selection Criteria

The number of proposed projects must be sufficient to allow the FUND to pick and choose the best A good ratio of applications to acceptances might be in the range of 10:1 Whereas commercial viability will constitute the first and foremost selection criterion, every effort would be made to select projects which have a strong development character, are environmentally friendly and/or involve production technologies which are deemed to be vital and critical to the recipient country's current socio-economic needs. Thus, preference would be given to sectors such as (a) food processing (b) Water purification, (c) renewable energy (d) agricultural development, and (e) light engineering. In all cases, the emphasis would be on cost-effective, labour-intensive production technologies.

The FUND's ability to divest itself of its participation at a profit will be the ultimate test of the FUND's success. Ideally, the FUND should be able to do this within a maximum of one or two years, so as to enable it to effectively cycle its resources to other equally meritorious projects.

Proposals for VENCAP's Organisational Structure

Besides being run by an experienced FUND manager, VENCAP would be assisted in its investment decisions by National Advisory Committees (NACs), which would be established in all participating LICs and would be composed of prominent business persons, professional men and women and financiers. These NACs would be chaired by an experienced consultant/consulting firm selected by the FUND. No member of the NAC having business or family links with the person or firm applying for equity finacing would participate in the evaluation procedure. VENCAP would be represented on the Boards of Directors of the firms in which it has acquired minority stakes through one or several members of the relevant NAC. The FUND itself would be run by a Board of Directors in which all of the major investors would be represented (and possibly some NGOs PVOs).

Follow-up

It is hoped that this article will provoke sufficient interest to justify the convening of an international meeting of aid agency officials and experts to study the ideas set forth above, so as to facilitate VENCAP's formal launching as an operative force. The need is there, the customer are there, the goodwill is there, only the financing and the organisation are lacking!

12

Richer or Poorer?

Achievements and Challenges of Ethical Trade

Ethical trade as an approach to supply chain management has mushroomed in recent years. Northern companies are becoming increasingly concerned with the 'ethics' of their operations and risks to reputation and productivity posed by bad employment practices in global supply chains. But can voluntary private sector codes really improve employment conditions in supply chains?

Ethical trade is one dimension of corporate social responsibility, bringing social issues into the mainstream of commercial supply chain management through the use of codes of conduct. It is sometimes confused with fair-trade which addresses terms of trading for smaller producers, and fosters greater responsibility in supply chain relations.

Ethical trade, on the other hand, focuses on workplace issues, requiring that supplier's in particular meet minimum employment, worker welfare and aspects of human rights standards.

Similar management systems are well established for product safety and environmental issues, Here we focus on the social dimensions of ethical trade and its codes of conduct yet the separation of social and environmental standards is increasingly artificial in global sourcing agreements. A plethora of codes are on of fer. The most numerous are in-houses codes such as Nike's 233 company codes counted in 1999 and the figure is rising.

Suppliers have to comply with and pay for multitude of similar but different codes. Harmonising codes or establishing equivalence is on the agenda but has not yet halted the problem of 'code overload'

At a broader level, industry-specific codes have also been developed. The US Apparel Industry Partnership/Fair Labour Agreement adopted by a number of leading US merchandising companies is a good example. Industry standards are not new, as ISO and EMAS environmental management systems show. Building on ISO principles, Social Accountability International (formerly CEPAA) has development SA8000. This is an independent social standard that can be used as an auditable code throughout the private sector.

Ethical trade is partly a response to consumer and campaigning group pressure in globalised economy. Alliances of companies, NGOs, trade. Developing codes of conduct through a multi stakeholder approach is a striking aspect of ethical trade, bringing together companies, NGOs, trade unions and some government departments. An example of this collaborative approach is the Ethical Trading Initiative (ETI) in the UK. The ETI's baseline code of conduct that corporate members from various industries must comply with as a minimum standard is more than just a code, ETI aims to provide a learning environment and sponsors pilot projects in developing countries to test different methods of monitoring and verification.

Codes of conduct need to be assessed in term of content, implantation and impact. A number of professional auditing companies have moved into his area, some accredited to audit specific codes such as FLA or SA8000. Suppliers audited against a specific code undergo an inspection, and where non-compliance is found, have to take remedial action or risk failing the audit.

Social auditing is a complex process, however, and it can be difficult to spot work place abuse, such as sexual harassment or force overtime, Workers have little confidence in a process that appears to be linked with management, and fear that reporting issues could risk their jobs. Advocates of the multi stakeholder approach argue that effective monitoring and verification of codes must involve local NGOs and trade unions in which workers have trust. Participatory social auditing also a means of raising awareness and of facilitating behavioral change, can help reveal serious management problems. But in many developing countries local organisations lack the capacity to participate: developing sustainable local systems of monitoring and verification remains an important challenge.

Do the advantages of multi-stakeholder approaches outweigh immediate constraints? Ethical trade is a largely northern driven process, reflecting Western ethical thinking and priorities, Southern based initiatives, however, are expanding, raising the possibility of local ownership of codes, collaboration poses challenges. Stronger relationships and better understanding are essential between southern and northern workers, producers, trade unions, and NGOs for codes to work globally.

But there is still scepticism as to the extent of the benefits that ethical trade might bring. Will increasing southern capacity to participate, as the ETI has done in its pilot project, help? Will building trust, confidence and dialogue achieve the objectives of ethical trade, north and south? Child labour is often more complex, however, than codes make it appear. Codes need to address the conditions of all workers within the supply chain, including the least visible; partnerships must include all groups to address these limitations.

The role of government is hotly contested. Can a system whose credibility depends on under-resourced civil society actors, often excluding democratically elected representatives, maintain genuine credibility? If the boundaries between private sector and public sector roles are not defined, the list of private sector responsibilities will become unmanageable. Private sector initiatives are not a substitute for more comprehensive national or international development policies.

What are the consequences of codes? Do they encourage downsizing or reinforce from large suppliers where compliance is more easily monitored? There is a risk that the gains of some will be at the expense of others.

Ethical trade has successfully begun forging partnerships to find solutions. While it might be wrong to assume that ethical trade can change the world, handled wisely it could make a world of difference for some. Yet it is not a panacea for development. Issues that remain unchallenged by ethical trade include:

- The exclusion of companies producing for domestic markets—often bigger employers.
- Underlying causes of poverty and social marginalisation.

13

The Challenges of Globalisation

Globalisation gives rise in some quarters to fears that can lead to suspicion, protectionism, and policies that are ultimately self-destructive. Such fears cannot be allowed to frustrate the great potential of a world in which countries drawing closer together. We believe that countries can face the challenges of globalisation positively, demanding as those challenges may be.

All countries can benefit from full participation in the world's markets, including its financial markets. Protectionist pressures must be resisted and reversed, and the principles of openness and mulilaterism promoted by the World Trade Organisation, the IMF, and the World Bank must be honoured. And financial market integration should be seen as a positive force: it offers access of global financial intermediation and a stimulus for more competitive and efficient domestic financial sectors; and it promotes efficiency and growth worldwide.

How encouraging it is, therefore, to see that so many developing countries in transition have been freeing up their trade and exchange systems within the framework of our structural adjustment programs.

No country can afford to forgo the benefits of integration into global market: the alternative is marginalisation and stagnation. But all countries must take the steps to minimize the associated risks. More than ever before, countries need tightly disciplined macro economic policies to maintain a stable environment for investors, whether domestic or foreign. And while foreign capital can be a useful—and sometimes vital complement to domestic saving, it is not a substitute for it: domestic saving remains the key to investment and sustainable growth. It is also clear that strong financial institutions are essential to avoid market disturbances at home and to secure an effective defense against external pressures. Competitive banking and financial systems that are sound, well regulated, and properly supervised are indispensable for countries to be able to expose their economies safely to the pressure that can arise in global markets.

The challenges to globalisation therefore add to the need for the developing and transition countries to press ahead with their adjustment and reform efforts. For many, this means creating conditions to attract foreign financing and use it effectively. But a growing number of countries have been facing a different problem: how to cope with large-scale capital inflows. Such inflows, especially when they are easily reversible; provide no grounds for relaxation of adjustment and reform.

They should not be used to finance domestic consumption. In many cases, they call for stronger fiscal discipline; and in some cases, exchange rates should be allowed to take part of the strain. Many developing countries and countries in transition also, of course, need to do more to deepen and widen the role of market forces and to foster more competitive market environments in order to promote transparent and efficient mechanisms of resource allocation.

Is globalisation any less demanding for the industrial countries? Not at all !It adds to the urgency of the task of taking full advantage of the current expansion to tackle the deep-rooted problems that are limiting the pace, the quality, and perhaps, the sustainability of their growth.

All has to applaud the increased efforts and commitments to reduce fiscal deficits, but in most cases underlying imbalances remain large and the pace of consolidation too slow. More must be done not only to redress present imbalances but also to meet the growing demands of the future.

Another deep-rooted problem-structural unemployment must also be tackled sooner, rather than later. Budget laxity and high unemployment tend to feed on each other. While cyclical conditions provide the opportunity, governments must not flinch from the task of improving the functioning of labor markets. How? It is not an easy task: by reforming regulations and policies that impede employment creation and job search.

Monetary stability, macroeconomic discipline, sound financial systems, and efficiently working market mechanisms are essential for all countries that embrace globalisation. But they are not sufficient for any. To fight the fears that globalisation sometimes inspires, countries need policies that promote not just economic efficiency, financial stability, and growth but also equity and high quality growth. In too many countries, the quality of growth suffers from widening distributional inequalities related partly to high unemployment but also stagnating wages of unskilled workers. And too many countries continue to suffer from poor governance, corruption and increasing crime.

Of course, economic policy can provide only part of what is needed to rid the world of these blights. But it is a vital part. To promote equity, efficiency, and sustainable growth, governments carry an inescapable responsibility for investment in human capital through education, health care, and well-targeted social safety nets - and also for establishing and maintaining honest and effective systems of public administration, law, order and justice. If these essential services are to be affordable, there is certainly no room for unproductive expenditures—military or otherwise—and wasteful subsidies: they must bear the brunt of fiscal consolidation. So globalisation demands a lot from governments if it is to deliver its promise of stronger and high-quality growth.

14

Few Signs of Hope in Africa

In 1996 a dozen countries in Africa achieved the targeted 6 per cent annual growth in gross domestic product (GDP), while the number of countries suffering from negative growth rates dropped from 19 in 1992 to three in 1996. These figures sound a lot less positive, however, if one compares GDP growth rates with population growth figures. Africa is still far ahead of other developing regions in the world in that respect and continues to grow at annual rates of 2.9 per cent. This means that the continent's estimated total population of 750 million (1996) will double to 1.5 billion by them year 2025. Whatever economic progress can be achieved until the, will have to be shared among an ever greater number of people. From 1991 to 1996 for instance, only 17 countries managed to expand their economies faster than their populations. In 35 countries, this was not the case. Their populations grew faster than their economic production or, in other words, even with modest economic advances, the population as a whole was worse off at the end of the period. On average, Africa's GDP grew by 2.3 per cent in 1996—not such a bad result when compared, for instance, with that of industrialised Europe. But when considering the 2.9 per cent population increase, the continent was left with an actual per capital income decline of 0.6 per cent.

If Africa wants to get out of this spiral of growing poverty, its government must do everything in their power to bring down the increase in their populations. However, a slow-down in population growth will not be enough to help Africa get out of its economic misery, especially since demographic changes are extremely weak as a partner in international economic relations, and the situation seems to be getting worse. Its share of world trade has fallen from 3.1 per cent in 1990 to 2.1 per cent in 1996. The continent still relies for its export earnings on a handful of primary commodities, among them oil, minerals, timber and agricultural goods. But the long term trend for these commodities is not very promising, given stiff competition from Asia and Latin America and slackening demand in industrial countries. World trade is no longer in commodities—their share in total exports dropped from 25.9 per cent (1990) to 19 per cent (1996). But Africa has not been able to keep up with its competitors from other developing countries who diversified their exports and trading partners and switched to the export of processed goods and manufactures.

The liberalisation of trade after the conclusion of the Uruguay Round is seen in Africa as a danger rather than a chance: estimates are that Africa will initially lose up to 3 billion dollars a year due to Uruguay, mainly from hikes in import bills, budget deficits, and the loss of preferences with the European Union. Unfortunately, the poor trade performance Africa on world markets is in no way compensated by trade among African countries. Despite numerous efforts in recent decades to promote intra-regional trade, poor roads, railways, waterways and communications have prevented any significant progress in this regard. One of the biggest obstacles to increased regional trade is lack in diversification, which the has resulted on too many countries producing the same or similar commodities.

When the New Africa Development Agenda was launched six years ago, the UN Secretary General has estimated that official development assistance (ODA) to Africa would have to be raised to 30 billion dollars for 1992, with a subsequent annual increase of 4 per cent. This target has proved to be illusionary. In actual fact, ODA barely reached 23.5 billion in 1995 and has continued to decline ever since. Although multilateral institutions increased their lending for Africa, the fall in bilateral funds could hardly be compensated.

Private finance also largely neglected Africa as a target for investments. In spite of the political and economic reforms implemented under structural adjustment programmes in no less than 37 African countries, entrepreneurs apparently found it safer and more profitable to invest their money in East Asia, Eastern Europe or Latin America. Of the 60 billion dollars in foreign direct investment (FDI) that went to developing countries in 1996, only 2.1 billion ended up in Africa. The share of the African continent in FDI dropped from 10 per cent (1987-91) to only 3.6 per cent now.

All these are rather depressing figures, which are hardly able to inspire new confidence in the future of the continent. One signal of hope, however, comes from the recent annual meeting of the International Monetary Fund and the World Bank in Washington. After protracted negotiations among creditor nations, an agreement has now been concluded to alleviate the debt burden of poor countries, many of them in Africa. The initiative which will lead to debt cancellations of some 7 billion dollars aims at bringing the debt service burden down to "sustainable" levels. Compared to the total indebtedness of Africa—which now stands at some 314 billion dollars—the amounts in question may seem insignificant. For some of the most heavily indebted countries, however, the scheme may provide the urgently needed breathing space, which will allow the benefiting country to make a new start.

The Midterm Review of progress achieved under Africa's New Development Agenda is anything but encouraging. The UN Secretary General has responded to the challenge by launching yet another effort—a Special Initiative on Africa—to mobilise support for the region. The special initiative is built on 20-priority action programmes focusing on water, basic education, health, and capacity building for governance and food security. Whether this programme will be able to attract more international support than its predecessors remains to be seen. More likely than not, the present international apathy concerning Africa's development will persist. It is ironical that the once much maligned Bretton Woods institutions are now the most reliable partners of Africa, while for bilateral donors, the continent is slowly drifting away.

15

Promotion of Industry and Foreign Investment in Africa

For more than a decade now industrialisation focusing on the promotion of private sector initiative and the encouragement of foreign investment has been given high rank in economic development policy by the authorities in most African countries. Yet, none of these have materialised with any significant impact in most of sub-Saharan Africa. Consequently, an atmosphere of general disappointment and even discouragement with African industrialisation is spreading, increasing some doubts whether adopted policies and programmes are worth-being pursued. This is certainly not a constructive environment and calls for a revision of assumptions, expectations and the means employed, in order to set more realistic and attainable prospects.

After independence, governments usually took a strong stand in regulating the economy and involved themselves in setting up and controlling a great number of state-owned enterprises. Preference was given to large and often capital-intensive enterprises either in production of basic consumer goods for the domestic markets or primary production and processing of export commodities. The role of private industry was relatively neglected or left without clear incentives to operate in the import substitution small and medium sized enterprises (SME) sector. A skeptical, sometimes hostile attitude prevailed towards foreign investment, which was usually controlled and regulated by restrictive concessions and investment laws.

In the early 1980s it had to be recongised that these policies were rather unsuccessful and could hardly be sustained. Growing budget deficits, high foreign debt and reduced flows of foreign credit imposed a revision of previous orientations. Structural adjustment policies were designed and gradually pursued. They basically implied:

- a general reduction of State control of economies;
- liberalisation of internal markets and opening to international competition;
- market adjustment of currency exchange mechanisms;
- deliberate opening to foreign investment;
- privatisation of State-owned enterprises and promotion of private enterprise in general.

Disappointing Results

However, what are the factual results to-date? Basically, all the global performance data show a rather bleak picture for sub-Saharan Africa in recent years, especially in comparison to other developing regions. Real annual GDP growth barely reached 1.5 per cent and growth of manufacturing industry has not significantly improved. Hence the GDP contribution of manufacturing industry remains below 15 per cent in most countries. Sub-Saharan Africa's share of total export volume stagnates and is the lowest of all developing regions. Exports continue to contain mostly primary commodities and only some 10 per cent of manufactured products. Compared with other regions, Africa continues with the lowest rate of private investment (some 8% of GDP in 1995) . Whereas Latin America and East Asia attract together about 80 per cent of net foreign direct investment to developing regions, the African share fluctuates between 1 and 2 per cent.

Constraints and Opportunities

The major constraints for advanced industrialisation in Africa can be briefly recalled.

Restricted Size of Domestic Markets

This is of prime importance for foreign investment which predominantly seeks access and expansion into new markets But also for local investors, it is a serious obstacle as certain technologies and industrial units need a substantial market size to achieve economies of scale. Regional market integration, often advocated as desirable solution, has not made significant progress for various, apparently quite persistent reasons (of which economic nationalism is one—and not only in Africa).

Comparatively High Factor Cost

Besides labour cost and productivity, which are not a decisive advantage in Africa in comparison to other developing regions, the shortage of skilled manpower with industrial experience, as well as infrastructural environment and logistics and generally a lack of integration (inter-sectoral linkage) are restricting factors.

Scarcity of Foreign Exchange

The general shortage of foreign exchange and the exchange rate fluctuations create major obstacles and uncertainties, especially for local market oriented industries which typically depend strongly on imported inputs. This also seriously restricts investment finance which often has to be contracted, and repaid, in foreign currency.

Lack of Financial Resources

Equity capital resources of African entrepreneurs are generally quite limited, and medium to long-term bank loans are constrained by low savings ratios and restrictive conditions of the banking sector.

Limiting Number of Industrial Entrepreneurs

Most entrepreneurs in African countries are found in the artisanal and small industry sector, whereas the small number of potential investors with the financial strength for medium to large enterprise comes from a trading and service background. The latter are usually led by a short-term profit motive and lack to some extent the relevant management experience for industrial enterprise.

Large-scale Enterprises with Investments above Some ECU 5 Million

If we call this category large, this of course is in relation to the context in most African countries: what is "large" there, might well be considered medium or small-sized from an industrialised country stand-point-and that is part of the dilemma. Typically, in this category, one finds mining and mineral exploitation companies, agricultural commodity production and primary processing enterprises, mostly geared towards export markets furthermore, some industries predominantly in food, beverages, textile and construction materials branches producing for local or sometimes regional markets.

The number of enterprises in this range is not more than a few dozens in most countries and only a few new investment opportunities are appearing or could be envisaged. This is rather a domain where many existing companies are State-owned and are seeking privatisation, or where some of the private-owned companies require rehabilitation and restructuring in order to face competitive market conditions.

With some exceptions there is a general tendency of multinational investors to get less involved in standard commodity production; and further processing of primary mineral and agricultural products is maintained closer to the markets in industrialised countries rather than being shifted to primary producing countries. Hence, for the traditional resource-based industries with export orientation, there will be some scope for quantitative expansion, but rather little real prospect for local further processing and linkage with domestic economies.

Large, local market-oriented enterprises will continue to be constrained by limited domestic purchasing power, lack of international competitiveness and a serious shortage of foreign exchange, the latter so much more when they require high import contents. There is usually little scope for a multiplication and diversification in this domain, as often one single enterprise unit covers the entire domestic demand (like petroleum refineries, cement factories, cereal mills, breweries, textile mills). If they present some attraction to private, also foreign investment, this still is often conditioned by protection allowing quasimonopolistic market positions.

Small and Medium-sized Enterprises (SMEs)

The great majority of manufacturing enterprises is in this category. It is basically composed of import substitution activities mostly for local consumer goods; some production and processing of local inputs for export (e.g. nontraditional agro products like vegetables and flowers, wood based products, processed fish) and some labour-intensive manufacturing, typically under free-zone status. There are only a few enterprises producing intermediate or investment goods for the local market (like metal and construction material industries).

As recently evidenced in several African countries (e.g. in Ghana, Zimbabwe and Uganda), considerable growth potential exists and some investment can be mobilised for SMEs. Non-traditional exports provide good opportunities, especially as they earn foreign exchange. Free-zone industries have some potential in selected countries, as already known from Mauritius and indicated by more recent trends e.g. in Madagascar and Cape Verde. But the core potential for SMEs remains probably in domestic markets, which involves the challenge for selective import substitution, where it can be efficient, and for the processing of local materials, with appropriate technologies and unit sizes for the basic local demand.

Perspectives for International Cooperation

Many of the leading multilateral and bi-lateral development institution have adopted policies and are providing programmes, mechanisms and resources to assist the development of industry in Africa, to facilitate private foreign investment as well as various forms of enterprise partnership. The World Bank Group has been particularly active in this domain by creating over the last ten years specialised facilities like the Foreign Investment Advisory Service (FIAS), the African Project Development Facility (APDF), the African Management Services company and the Africa Enterprise Fund (AEF) through which the International Finance Corporation provides direct investment funding to medium-sized companies. The European Union put strong emphasis on private enterprise and investment in the fourth Lome Convention and besides institutional assistance towards a better legislative and administrative environment, offers a comprehensive range of financial and technical support to enterprises. The number of projects implemented by the European Commission, especially geared to small-scale industry by way of technical assistance, credit lines and guarantee funds has grown significantly.

Financial resources managed by the EIB, especially risk capital provided from the European Development Fund, were strongly increased and a significant portion has been devoted to investment in the private sector. Some new mechanisms were introduced to make the use of risk capital more flexible and suitable for direct financing of larger projects and indirect financing of SMEs via local credit institutions. The Centre for the Development of Industry (CDI) has been strengthened for its tasks to promote EU-ACP enterprise partnerships and to support the creation or improvement of SMEs. It is noteworthy that CDI can offer its range of practical services directly to individual investors and existing enterprises.

Hence it appears that, although private foreign investors for Africa are scarce, there is no scarcity of external means and mechanisms to assist African enterprise. Yet there is probably a need to better adapt the means to prevailing conditions, to orientate them with clearer priorities towards effective growth potentials and to coordinate them for higher efficiency.

16

Crisis and New Orientation of Development Policy

The poverty in the South, the dislocations in the East, and the orientation crisis in the North are not isolated phenomena. Rather, they represent an alarming amalgamation of dangers that are globally interlinked.

The low effectiveness of international economic and development policy is rooted in two outdated paradigms on which the present worldwide strategy of economic development is based, namely that:

1. The Western social and economic model optimizes the activation of productive forces—independent of the development stage of a country and its culture and therefore is best suited to satisfy basic needs.

2. It is possible to launch the development of a society from the outside within a few decades-without regard to its cultural and historical background—through external input of money, goods, technology, expertise, and personnel.

The twin paradigms of the timelessness and transferability combined with cultural ecological, and financial restrictions—have led international cooperation and development down the wrong path.

Only if we acknowledge the true dimensions of the global dangers, if we recognise the limitations and shortcomings of existing political instruments, and identify outdated theories and contradictory special interests, can we outline the cornerstones of a new policy of global cooperation.

Cornerstones of a New Development Policy

Starting with critical review of the shortcomings and paradigms of the prevailing development strategy, the following ten cornerstones of a new development policy are offered for discussion:

1. Broaden the Concept of Development

Whether a society is considered developed depends on the size of its percapita Gross National Product (GNP). Accordingly, the world is divided into a developed, semi-developed, and underdeveloped world. The yardstick for development, which has become the norm in the industrial countries, is one-dimensional: It only measures the monetary value of goods and services that are exchanged in the marketplace. This standard is too narrow economically because, it compresses the multitude and complexity of cultural, societal historical, social, and human values into a single economic category.

At the most, there can and should be agreement on what development and process should not bring about: Inability to find enough work to meet the most basic needs; exploitation and oppression of people; loss of cultural wealth and institutions; destruction of natural resources. These, however, are the very values that are scarified by the prevailing development strategy. In the future, development policy must do all it can to stop the loss of skills and self-reliance, the plunder of natural resources, the erosion of cultural values, the violation of human dignity and human rights. Initiatives must prevail which are orientated on these values, and not just on the GNP.

2. Concentrate Development Strategy on the Internal Potential of Developing Countries

There must be an end to the manic fixation of development strategy on external inputs and external markets. A new development policy must, above all, improve internal conditions for a productive economy, promote domestic production factors on a broad basis, protect cultural and natural resources, and greatly increase the domestic supply of basic goods. Wherever external inputs are unavoidable, credits must be strictly tied to the productivity and the ability of a country to absorb transfers. External transfers should be concentrated on "Software" for health, education, and social participation, administrative, and legal jurisdiction. Such an approach could also promote training and indigenous technologies, which are so important for economic development.

The set-up and expansion of the productive sectors must be decided, planned, and implemented by the developing countries themselves, and they must assume full responsibility. The external pressures, which force the developing countries into full integration with the world market, must be removed. This presupposes a structural reduction of interest rates.

3. *Make Development Policy a Central Feature of Polities*

Development policy must take the lead in mobilizing the various political forces and government departments to join the fight against the growing global dangers. It must ensure that the actions of all political departments are compatible with development policy is possible only if it becomes the central task of all political sectors, comparable to social and environmental policies, and the central goal of all policies. If development policy is to become a central task, development problems must become a priority in parliament and government. Society must understand that it is in the national interest to accept great global responsibilities.

4. *Reform the World Economy*

The industrial countries must abolish their protectionism in agriculture as well the processed goods sector. Simultaneously, the developing countries need to be protected selectively and for a limited time against imports from the industrial countries. The undifferentiated structural adjustment policies imposed by the IMF must be revised. The trend toward regionalisation of the world economy should not be opposed; rather, in the interest of both South and East, it must be regulated constructively to form a new, regionally based world trade structure.

A reform of the international finance system is urgently needed: Interest and exchange rates should not mirror the national interests of the big industrial states and the special interests of large banks and venture capital. Rather, they must reflect the global interest in monetary stability lower and stable interest rates, and sufficient development financing.

However, strengthening the international financial institutions is in the global interest only if the countries of the southern and eastern hemispheres are allowed to exert some influence. An international financial court must guarantee that violations of strict regulations to ensure international stability and solvency can be protested in a court of law.

5. *Redesign the Industrial Society*

As a global social and environmental policy, the new development policy must induce the industrial countries to give up their excessive consumption of air, water, soil, resources, and space. Increased utilisation of energy-conservation measures and environmentally friendly technologies is overdue. The economic and social policies of the industrial nations must promote balance rather than growth. This requires radical changes in traditional economic thinking, habits, structures and processes.

In view of limited world resources, unsatisfied existential needs in South and East, and continuous population growth in the south, the only premise for the future can be: Growth rates in the South must be higher than in the North, but they should no longer be in the North, but they should no longer be induced primarily by growth in the North. If economic policies continue to call for the North to provide the locomotive, the North will have to continue to acquire more resources than the south.

The North must relinquish the remaining growth frontiers to the South and East. The South must use this opportunity to activate its internal dynamic potential rather than integrate its economy with the North. However, ecological and social controls must be established at a much earlier stage than was the case in Europe.

6. *Strengthen Development Cooperation*

The share of official development assistance as a percentage of GNP, which dropped from 0.48 per cent in 1982 to 0.34 per cent in 1995 must be gradually raised again and reach at least 0.7 per cent in the year 2000—a goal which OECD established as early as two decades ago and which was reconfirmed at the Rio Earth Summit.

However, we must not succumb to the illusion that a doubling of ODA funds will even remotely meet the financial needs of South and East. State development policy must use it scarce public funds more effectively in the future. It must use restraint whenever partners in the developing countries can accomplish a task on their own and private initiatives and private enterprise are more competent to do the job. The government should be directly engaged only when it can be relatively more productive. Otherwise, it should limit itself to subsidizing private organisations.

7. *Now Orientation for Development Cooperation*

The state and its implementation agencies must abandon all direct responsibility for any projects which require unbureaucratic action, economic efficiency, and long term productivity. It must make a much greater effort to involve NGO's and private venture capital in development projects. At the same time, the state must insist and guarantee that private actions are compatible with social and ecological concerns.

In the future, the main thrust of government projects should be the promotion of the internal potential of a country. This comprises the political and administrative framework conditions of a humane, socially and ecologically sound development: Constitutional government, social institutions which facilitate broad participation of the population in politics, society, and economy; efficient savings, credit fiscal and financial systems; mechanisms for income, property, and land distribution which, promote productivity, justice, and social peace. In additional of this "software" of development, the following is needed: A regimen for the protection of resources and environment; measures to prevent the short term sellout of natural resources; elementary and general education and training, health care and social safety nets; capacities to develop science and technology.

8. *Reduce the Debt Service and Activate Private Capital*

Public funds must be used be to a greater degree for the financial rehabilitation of highly indebted countries in South and East; external demands for interest and principal payments must be adapted to the economic capacity of the respective country and its ability to execute external capital transfers.

Within the framework of international insolvency regulations, initiatives must be developed as condition for the continuance of the present rules for write-offs—which ensure effective cooperation from the banks and alleviate the heavy burden of private credits, with their high interest rates.

State development policy and private business interests should supplement each other. Government promotion of private enterprise initiatives for exports, investment, and employment in the developing countries must take into account their compatibility with development. In reverse, private engagements that effectively promote development must be actively supported by the government. A separate line item must be established in the development budget for such activation of private capital

9. *Set Regional Priorities*

State development cooperation has been scattering its scarce funds that not only among too many sectors, but also among too many partners. In the future, public funds must be concentrated regionally. More emphasis must be placed on regional programmes, and development cooperation with threshold countries must be enhanced. A portion of public funds should be set aside to provide an incentive for be set aside to provide an incentive for threshold countries to assist the poorer nations in their own region as well as deal with poverty in their own country.

The new development policy could then also help lessen ethnic-national conflicts and promote peace by sponsoring regional cooperation in joint development projects. For this purpose, regional development funds must be set up for cooperation in the transportation, energy, trade, and finance sectors and last, but not least for regional security systems and disarmament. Such regional funds could also provide the means to project refugees and improve their prospects for an eventual return to their homelands.

Food Security:

Availability and Access to Food

The world food situation has never been better. Enough food is being produced today that, if it were evenly distributed, no one should have to go hungry. World food production is increasing faster than population growth: per capital production increased by 5 per cent during the 1980s. Real food prices are at historic lows and have been declining for some time now. Yields of major cereals have more than doubled in the past three decades. These trends have contributed to complacency in some quarters regarding the world food situation.

Yet, more than 700 million people in the developing world do not have access to sufficient food to lead healthy and productive lives. More than 180 million children are underweight. Diseases of hunger and malnutrition are widespread. The desire to satisfy food needs has, in combination with increasing population densities and inadequate agricultural intensification, led to much degradation of environmentally fragile lands, such as foress and steep hillsides.

Over the next 20-30 years, farmers and policy makers in developing countries will be challenged to provide food at affordable prices for almost 100 million more people every year—the largest annual population increase in history. Moreover, they will have to increase food production from more productive use of the land and without further degradation of natural resources: area expansion is no longer a feasible option in most of the world.

What future food security will look like depends not on exogenous factors over which we have no control but on the decisions and actions taken by the major players: households, privates and public sector agencies, governments, and the international community. If we continue to act as we have in the 1980s and early 1990s, more people will suffer from food insecurity it will be because some or all of these players failed to at in an appropriate and timely manner.

Feeding the World: Availability and Access to Food

There is enough food in the world today to feed everyone, if it were evenly distributed. Availability of daily food energy per capita in the developing countries as a whole increased by 0.7 per cent per year during the 1980s.

Twenty-five developing countries, including about half of the African countries, were unable to assure sufficient food energy (2,200 calories per person per day) for their populations at the end of the 1980s even if available food energy were evenly distributed within each country. This is down from 45 countries at the end of the 1970s.

However, available food is neither evenly distributed nor fully consumed. Availability of enough food at global, regional, or national levels does not necessarily mean that everyone is well fed. For people to be food secure—that is, to have access at all times to the food required for a healthy and productive life—there must be both availability of food and access to food. Access to food by households (and individuals) is conditioned by poverty: the poor usually lack adequate means to secure access to food.

Over 1.1 billion people in developing countries were living in poverty in 1993, more than 500 million in conditions of extreme poverty. South Asia is the home of about 50 per cent of the developing world's poor—more than 500 million people. Another 15 per cent are found in East Asia, 19 per cent in sub-Saharan Africa, and 10 per cent in Latin America and the Caribbean. The prevalence of poverty (the proportion of each region's population that is poor) is very high—about 50 per cent—in South Asia as well as in sub-Saharan Africa.

Today, there are more than 700 million people who do not have access to sufficient food to meet their needs for a healthy and productive life; they often go hungry adults and children also suffer from diseases associated with hunger and poverty. For almost one fifth of the total population of developing countries to be chronically hungry tarnishes the images of a world that is now considered food-secure because it produces enough food.

Great progress has been made in meeting food needs during the last 30 years. For instance, the number of underfed people declined from an estimated 976 million in 1974-76 to 786 million in late 1980s. But the problem is far from solved. Keeping up with increasing needs and demands due to population growth, income increases, and dietary changes is itself a formidable challenge.

Hunger and food insecurity have a significant effect on health and nutrition of both adults and children. They can lead to growth failure in children. About 184 million pre-school children in developing countries were underweight in 1994. About 55 per cent of these underweight children were found in South Asia and another 16 per cent in sub-Saharan Africa. The proportion of children that are underweight is higher in South Asia (almost 60 per cent), but it is also significant in Sub-Saharan Africa (30 per cent) and Southeast Asia (31 per cent). It is worrisome that the number of underweight children in Sub-Saharan Africa during the 1980s from 20 million to 28 million is particularly striking.

In addition to energy deficiencies, micro nutrient deficiencies are also widespread in the developing world. About 14 million pre-school children (under the age of five years) have eye damage as a result of Vitamin-A deficiency. Ten million of these children are found in Southeast Asia. Between 250,000 and 500,000 pre-school children go blind each year due to Vitamin-A deficiency, two-thirds of these children die within months of going blind. Many more children are mildly affected. Recently research has shown that even mild deficiencies can increase mortality significantly. Vitamin-A deficiencies are closely linked to diet, which can be influenced by agricultural research and policy.

Iron deficiency affects about 1 billion people in the world. particularly children and women of reproductive age. Iron deficiency leads to anaemia, which if not checked can diminish learning capacity and increase morbidity and morality. In the developing countries, about 370 million women between 15 and 49 years of age—42 per cent of this population group—where anaemic in the 1980s. Almost one-half were in South Asia. And there are tentative indications from South Asia and sub-Saharan Africa that the prevalence of anaemia is rising in non pregnant adult women of reproductive ages.

In sub-Saharan Africa, this trend is undoubtedly associated with deterioration in general standards of living, including increased poverty and food insecurity. Anaemia partly arises from diets insufficient in iron, which again could be addressed through agricultural research and policy. For example, a possible reason why iron deficiency and anaemia are going up in South Asia may lie in the decrease in production of iron rich pulses during that same period, which in part reflects the larger research input into competing crops such as wheat in South Asia. This emphasizes the importance of considering the effects on diet and thus on health and nutrition in setting research priorities for yield-increasing research.

South Asia is the home of about half of the developing world's hungry and food-insecure people, but this population group is growing rapidly in sub-Saharan Africa. Much of the poverty and food insecurity is in rural areas, mainly in low-potential areas such as arid zones, but urban poverty is also growing rapidly.

Four Key Factors will Influence Future Food Production and Consumption

Global and regional food production and consumption during the next 10-20 years will be influenced by a large number of factors. Changes in the following four sets of factors are likely to particularly important:

1. Economic growth and economic policies;
2. Population growth and urbanisation;
3. Rural infrastructure, agricultural production technology, and access to modern inputs; and
4. Natural resource management and environmental consideration.

The expected impact of each of these factors on future food production and consumption is considerable.

Economic Growth and Economic Policies

Economic growth must resume in the developing world, especially in Sub-Saharan Africa. To support such growth, it is critical to:

- complete structural adjustment and economic reforms;
- remove external barriers to growth such as trade distortions and subsidies in developed countries;
- liberalize trade and remove market distortions;
- enhance access by the poor to land, capital, and technology;
- expand investment in rural infrastructure, health, education, and agricultural research and technology;
- facilitate sustain ability in agricultural production; and
- reverse the decline in international assistance to agriculture.

Growth in real per capita income during the 1980s was disappointing for developing countries as a whole. However, the low average rate of growth covers large variations among regions. The high rates of economic growth in Asia are expected to continue through the 1990s, while incomes in Sub-Saharan Africa are expected to keep pace with population growth.

Future economic growth depends on internal policies as well as on the international policies as well as on the international environment. The extent to which current structural adjustment and economic reforms in Latin America, Sub-Saharan Africa, the Commonwealth of Independent States (CIS), Eastern Europe, and selected countries in Asia and the Middle East are carried to successful completion at an appropriate speed and sequence is of paramount importance for future economic growth in those countries.

Closely related to this issue is the question of the most appropriate role of the stable in a market-oriented economy with inappropriate institutions, poor infrastructure, and insufficient experience by the private sector in dealing effectively in a competitive market environment. Overreaction to past failures such as excessive and inappropriate state intervention may cause governments to take on a passive role where intervention is needed to assure that the markets function effectively and to deal with outside influences on the economy.

Future economic growth will also depend on the international trade environment, including trade distortions by developed countries, and access to external aid. Import restrictions for agricultural and non-agricultural products in Japan, the European Union, and the United States, along with domestic agricultural subsidies and implicit and explicit export subsidies for agricultural products, are of particular concern.

Population Growth and Urbanisation

If progress in economic growth is not to be undermined by rapid population growth and excessive urbanisation, effective population and migration policies are necessary to complement growth-oriented policies. Such policies must focus on:

- universal access to family planning information and technology; and
- incentives to reduce rural-urban migration, such as provision of employment in rural areas and stimulation of agricultural and non-agricultural growth in rural areas.

Although the annual growth rate is falling for the world as a whole, the population increase during the next 20-30 years, of slightly less than 100 million people a year, will be the largest ever. Approximately 97 per cent of this increase is projected to occur in the Third World, with Africa alone accounting for 34 per cent of the growth. Thus although reductions in annual population growth rates have begun to occur in Asia and Latin America, they are insufficient to counter the absolute increases. Population growth rates of these magnitudes will greatly increase the need for food and other basic necessities.

Rural Infrastructure, Agricultural Production Technology, and Access to Modern Inputs

Continued progress in all three of these areas is critical to future food security.

- Resources must be committed to infrastructure construction and maintenance. Labour-intensive public works programmes are a viable mechanisms for building roads, reforesting areas, and engaging in soil conservation projects, while creating employment and income in rural areas.
- International and national agricultural research must continue to develop yield-enhancing production technology, especially in maize, millet, and other crops, as well as build tolerance or resistance in crops to pests and adverse climatic conditions.
- Farmer access to modern inputs must be facilitated through provision of credit and technical assistance. Inputs must be made available to all farmers on time and in required amounts.

The importance of investments in rural infrastructure within the context of rapid urbanisation has already been established. Even without rapid urban growth, however, such investments are needed in many developing countries, particularly the poorest ones, to facilitate agricultural and rural development. Improved rural infrastructure enhances access to export markets, modern production inputs, and consumer goods. It reduces marketing costs, promotes exchange between intracountry markets, reduces spatial and temporal price distortions, and, in general, increases efficiency in production and marketing.

However, while essential, effective rural infrastructure alone is not enough to assure agricultural and rural development and rapid increases in food production in developing countries. Yield enhancing production technology is of critical importance. Although opportunities for expansion of agricultural production into lands not currently under cultivation still exist in some countries, such opportunities are so limited that they would probably not be able to counter losses of current agricultural lands to alternative uses on a global level. Furthermore, attempts to expand agricultural production into new lands would, in most cases, require large investments in technology, tools and materials and would increase the risk of land degradation and deforestation. Thus, future increases in food production must come primarily from higher yields per unit of land rather than from land expansion.

Agricultural research has successfully developed yield-enhancing technology for the majority of crops grown in temperate zones and for several crops grown in tropical zones. The dramatic impact of agricultural research and modern technology on wheat and rice yields in Asia and Latin American since the mid-1980s is well known. Less dramatic but significant yield gains have been obtained from research and technological change in other crops, particularly maize.

Natural Resource Management and Environmental Considerations

Research, technology development, incentives, and regulations are needed to prevent environmental degradation. These measures include appropriate water management policies, reduction of subsidies that encourage wasteful use of inputs better definition of ownership and user rights to resources including land, education of farmers to encourage appropriate use of technology and resource conservation, and the provision of alternatives to resource-degrading inputs and techniques. Since poverty is a major source of degradation, poverty eradication is justified also on environmental grounds.

The recent surge in public and private concerns about negative environmental effects of economic growth and development may, if sustained, have important implications for agricultural development and future food production and consumption. Of particular concern of the need to avoid degradation of natural resources such as land and water, as well as deforestation, water contamination, and health risks associated with the use of chemicals. Since most of the current and potential resource degradation and environmental contamination result from situations in which those who cause and possibly benefit from degradation do not pay the costs, neither the market nor the individual producers and consumers are likely to incorporate preventive measures into their behaviour. Only when sufficient damage has been done to influence significantly current or future production costs will market and producer behaviour change. The state is more likely to undertake preventive measures either through publicly funded research and technology development or through incentive policies and regulations. Extensive water logging, salination, and associated land degradation and productivity losses resulting from inappropriate water management are of particular concern in large parts of Asia.

No Time for Complacency

Population growth will outstrip growth in food production in Sub-Saharan Africa for a long time to come unless more is done to accelerate agricultural growth. Between now and 2000, the population will grow at more than 3 per cent a year, while food production is likely to grow at 2 per cent or less a year. By the year 2000, the production shortfall is estimated to increase to about 50 million tons of grain equivalent, up from the current level of about 14 million tons. The region will not have the necessary foreign exchange to import such large amounts of food. And Africa governments will not be able to count on enough food aid to make up the difference. If current trends continue, by the year 2020, Africa will have a food shortage of 250 million tons, which is more than 20 times the current food gap.

Poverty is expected to increase rapidly in the coming years. Sub-Saharan Africa's share of the world's poor is expected to increase from the current 19 per cent to about 28 per cent in 2000. Furthermore, the number of underweight children in expected to increase in the 1990's in Sub-Saharan Africa.

Asian demand for cereals is estimated to grow at an annual rate of 2.1 per cent between now and the year 2000, where as food production is expected to grow at 1.9 per cent per year. Much of the production shortfall is likely to be dealt with through expanded imports and perhaps through expanded regional production in response to price increases.

In Latin America, by contrast, growth in food production is anticipated to exceed food demand growth: food production is estimated to grow by 3 per cent annually between 1990 and 2000, while food demand is estimated to grow by 2.5 per cent per year.

Large areas of land are rapidly being degraded and deforested. And the principal reasons for environmental degradation—poverty, high population growth, and limited access to appropriate agricultural technology—are not being dealt with effectively.

About 700 million people are food insecure for them the food crisis has arrived. For the 10-12 million preschool children who died in 1994 from hunger and diseases related to malnutrition, the food crisis came and went. One-third of the preschool children of the Third World are unable to grow to their full potential and face increased risk of death and disease.

Complacency is not in order. Clearly, Mathus underestimated the power of science to expand food production. The mass starvation that was predicted the Asia in the 1970s and 1980s did not occur because science was effectively put to work to expand crop yields. However, past yield increases came about people with foresight made appropriate decisions. The failure to expand investments in agricultural research and technology development during the

1980s and 1990s indicates that such foresight no longer prevails. Given the long lag time between investment in agricultural research and the resulting production increases, failure to invest today will show up in production shortfalls 10 to 20 years from now. The problems associated with environmental degradation will present themselves sooner. We must not wait until a global food crisis is upon us or until the last tree has fallen to make these investments.

REFERENCES

1. FAO, FAO Production Yearbook.
2. FAO, "The State of Food and Agriculture 1992".
3. FAO, "Agriculture Towards 2010".
4. FAO, "The State of Food and Agriculture 1994".
5. FAO, Food Outlook (December 1994).
6. World Bank, World Development Report 1995.
7. World Bank, Global Economic Prospects and the Developing Countries.
8. World Food Programme, Food Aid in Review (Rome WFP 1992).
9. World Bank, Global Economic Prospects and the Development Countries 1992. (Washington, D.C.: World Bank).

18

Food First

By the time this day is over, about 40,000 human begins—Mostly children—will have died from hunger, malnutrition and related causes. Today and everyday the deaths will mount, reaching an annual toll of 13 to 18 million. Few of these people will have been caught up in famine or other emergencies. Most will have suffered from a "silent" assault—the kind that seldom makes the headlines, but which claims its victims just as relentlessly.

It is intolerable that such deprivation and suffering should be allowed to exist in a world of potential food plenty. Having enough food is fundamental to all else. At the most basic level, this may entail humanitarian relief to assist people in emergency situations. In the transition from relief to development, however, we must look at systems for ensuring that societies have the capacity to produce or purchase the food they need and that it is accessible to all.

Sustainable food security fuses the goals of household food security and sustainable agriculture; it requires both. It requires looking not only at the aggregate supply of food, but also at the distribution of income and land, and at other issues: Do people have enough income to buy food? Enough land to grow their own food? Does the food distribution system deliver food where it is needed? How much food is wasted due to inadequate distribution systems? What are the implications of trends in population growth for future food needs? What is the status of women in society, and what opportunities do women have to alter rapid population growth rates? What is being done to regenerate the resource base for food production? These questions need to be asked and answered in every country.

The challenge of sustainable food security is immense, and it is growing. One billion people—20 per cent of the global population—are too poor to obtain enough food to sustain normal work. Half a billion are too poor to obtain the food needed for healthy growth of children and minimal activity of adults. Today's failure to feed people, however, may be but a prologue to a much larger failure in the future. Given likely population increases, world food output must triple over the next 50 years if the world's people are to have a nutritionally adequate diet. It will be difficult enough to achieve this expansion under favourable circumstances, and conditions may be far from favourable.

For example, according to recent estimates an area of about 1.2 billion hectares—the size of China and India combined—has experienced moderate to extreme soil deterioration since World War II as a result of human activities. Over three-fourths of that deterioration has occurred in the developing regions from causes such as overgrazing, deforestation, land clearing, unsound agricultural practices and increased soil salinity and water logging, largely from irrigation. Other environmental threats to the agricultural resource base include loss of water and genetic resources, adverse effects of pesticides and climate change, both local and global.

At the most aggregate level, the required increase in food production could be met if production grew at the historic average, that is, at the two per cent per annum rate achieved over the past half-century. But is this realistic? To produce three times more calories, all the land currently under cultivation around the world would, within 50 years, have to attain levels of productivity as high as those exhibited by the very best cropland today.

To this challenge add the possibility of diminished returns from the technological, energy and other inputs that have made agriculture so successful. Some experts believe that most of the potential for increased output of cereals—from improved plant varieties, from increased use of pesticides and fertilizers and from expanding the area under irrigation—has already been captured.

Viewed from this perspective, the goal of achieving sustainable food security in the decades ahead emerges as one of the greatest challenges humanity has ever faced. Agricultural output must be tripled, and people must have the income to buy the food they need. The erosion of the resource base must be halted and then reversed. Failure on any of these fronts will yield unprecedented human suffering.

What will it take to achieve sustainable food security? Obviously, the effort will have to be immense, both in size and complexity. Outlined below are a few simple (but no easy) steps that are absolutely essential elements of serious effort.

First, as citizens of the world, we must all come to see sustainable food security as a fundamental aspect of global peace and human security. This goes well beyond merely denouncing the use of food as a weapon.

Second, we must adopt concrete international goals, such as reducing world hunger by half over the next 10 years. We will never achieve the goal of sustainable food security unless we aim at specific milestones, and assess rigorously our progress in moving toward them.

Third, we must forge a true global partnership, a compact for sustainable food security. All countries—rich and poor—have important roles and responsibilities. There must be reciprocal responsibilities among nations, not one-way transfers.

Fourth, we must see deterioration of the agricultural resource base—terrestrial, aquatic and climatic—for what it is: a major threat to development and a major source of economic loss. Farmers are the largest group of environmental decision-makers in the world. We must ensure that they have the means to make sustainable development a reality where it counts—in the fields and fisheries.

Fifth, we must empower the people who work the land and who keep it productive. They are in the best position to decide the most appropriate ways to graft new technology onto their own traditional knowledge of seed selection, plant protection and nutrient-cycling. Special emphasis should be given to the role of women, the main providers for two-thirds of the poorest households in the developing world, as well as the producers of 60 per cent of all food grown and consumed locally.

Sixth, we must build the capacities of developing countries, both in government and in civil society. Capacity-building means empowerment for self-reliance. It means strengthening national capacities, both inside and outside government. This is essential for recognition and analysis of problems, for decision-making on courses of action and for management of systems and processes.

Seventh, not only must we build capacity in developing countries, we must also create linkages among researchers in industrial and developing countries. This will help minimize the time lag between discovery and practical utilisation. In addition, analysts from various countries must work together to examine future food security issues with different scenarios of population growth, agricultural productivity, markets and trade, climate change, loss of soil and bio-diversity and, last but not least, political instability, in order to devise options for rational choices.

We know a good deal about how to rid the world of the scourge of hunger, and how to begin to move toward sustainable food security on a global basis. We know that economic growth and prosperity are necessary, though not sufficient, conditions for eradicating hunger. We also know that developing efforts must encompass not only food production, but also socio-economic factors, including sustainable livelihoods for poor families, the implications of population growth rates, the status of women and girls and so forth. We also know that good words are not enough. Now more than ever before it is crucial that we marshal the political will to achieve our goals.

19

Food for the Billions

Will there be enough food to feed 8 billion people who will live on earth in 25 years' time? Surprisingly few people, at least in the industrial countries, seems to be overly concerned with this question. Whereas the world conferences on the environment, on women, human rights or social issues which were held in recent years were preceded and accompanied by intensive public debate, food does not seem to be a burning issue. Don't we have mountains of surplus food, people ask. Do we not have to pay our farmers to leave their land idle in order not to add to the glut on the world markets? And hasn't the Green Revolution ended famine even in countries like India which used to be a synonym for hungry people? So where is the problem?

The advance made in agricultural production since beginning against a background of imminent crisis are indeed remarkable. In only 20 years, yields of major crops like rice, maize and wheat in developing countries went up by 80 per cent, outpacing even the rapid increase in population. But this growth in yields has slowed down in recent years, and the aim of "food for all" is once again becoming elusive. About 800 million people still do not have access to enough food to meet their basic daily needs, nearly 200 million children suffer from protein and energy deficiencies, 88 countries—44 of them in Africa—have a deficit in food production.

Everyone wants to increase food security. The definition is that "food be available at all times, that all persons have means of access to it, that it be nutritionally adequate in terms of quantity, quality and variety, and that it be acceptable within the given culture". To achieve this goal, more food must be produced—much more, because we must not only adequately feed the 5.8 billion people already on earth, but also the additional two billion who will be added to world population in the next 25 years. Critics argue that the problem is not one of production alone, but one of poverty elimination. People are not hungry because there is no food, but because they have no money to buy it, these critics say. Available resources must be better distributed to end hunger in the world.

However, even if we succeed to eliminate poverty in the next few decades—a feat which appears highly unlikely—there would still be the need to boost production, because with rising incomes people also want to eat more and better food including meat. As can already be observed in the countries of East Asia, the newly acquired wealth leads to higher consumption levels which puts additional strains on available resources are getting scarcer. Agricultural lands are being degraded at alarming speed by erosion, salinity, desertification or disappear altogether due to urban or infrastructure development. It has been estimated that 40 per cent of productive land now has diminished capacity to supply benefits to humanity due to direct human impacts of land use. Water for agricultural purposes is getting scarcer almost everywhere, and there are hardly any land reserves to be brought into production to widen the agricultural base.

In this situation, there is no alternative to increasing and improving production from the existing land area. This can only be done through research which finds the best varieties which will bring the highest yields at the lower cost to the environment. Sustainable agriculture is the key notion—one that maintains bio-diversity, uses as little chemical inputs as possible and does not over exploit water and soil resources.

In recent years, agricultural research has been neglected partly because of the erroneous belief that with mountains of meat and lakes of milk further production increases were not desirable. Since global grain production has stagnated and world stocks have reached an alarmingly low level last year, there has been a noticeable change of mind. To raise the awareness among governments around the world that promotion of agriculture is urgent if hunger is to be avoided in the next century.

Important work is already being done by the international agricultural research institutes which promoted the Green Revolution in the sixties and seventies and are now again in the forefront of finding solutions to the daunting task of feeding 8 billion people by the year 2020. The International Rice Research Institute (IRRI) in the Philippines, the Maize and Wheat Research Institute (CIMMYT) in Mexico or institutes like ICARDA in Syria and ICRISAT in India which work on agriculture in semi-arid and dry areas, are all seeking solutions to the problem of raising production while at the same time preserving the environment. These institutions as well as national agricultural research institutions need all the support from the public and, of course, appropriate funding, to help them accomplish their task.

The scientists are optimistic that they can develop the varieties and farming systems which will allow mankind to feed everyone on earth well into the next century. But the task is not for the scientists alone. An economic and political order must also be in place which makes it possible to eradicate poverty and allow everyone to enjoy the benefits that science can offer. Feeding the billions is, therefore not only a scientific, but first and foremost a political.

20

Food Production

During the last 25 years, world agriculture successfully expanded food production faster than population growth. This can continue for the next 25 years and beyond, if appropriate action is taken. Although world food stocks are currently low and grain prices high, the world is not about to run out of food. We can produce enough food for future generation if we choose to do so.

The widespread food insecurity, unhealthy living conditions, and abject and absolute poverty in many developing countries are already threatening global stability. Failure to assure sustainable food security will foster the very conditions that will further destabilise and polarise the world in the year to come with tremendous consequences for all people.

The Basic Facts

Poverty is widespread in developing countries, with over 1.1 billion people living on a dollar a day or less per person. Human resource development in developing countries is lagging: 1 billion people lack access to health services, 1.3 billion do not have access to adequate sanitation systems, and one-third of primary school enrolls drop out by Grade 4. Natural resources, upon which future food production depends, are being degraded at alarming rates: almost 2 billion hectares of land have been degraded in the past 50 years: about 180 million hectares of forests have been converted to other uses during the 1980s, marine fisheries are collapsing around the world, and regional and seasonal water shortage afflict many developing countries. Improved appropriate technology is essential to increase productivity. Yet low-income food deficit developing countries are grossly under investing in agricultural research and many are reducing their support.

It calls for sustained action in six priority areas. First, we must selectively strengthen the capacity of developing country governments to perform appropriate functions such as establishing or clarifying property rights, promoting private-sector competition in agricultural markets, and maintaining appropriate macro economic environments. Predictability, transparency and continuity in policy making and enforcement must be pursued.

Investing in People

Second, we must invest more in poor people in order to enhance their productivity, health, and nutrition. It is not only unethical but economically wasteful that a large share of the world's population is malnourished, illiterate, sick, and without access to productive resources. Access to primary education, primary health care, reproductive care and family planning information, and clean water and sanitation must be assured for all people. Access by the poor to productive resources and remunerative employment must be improved. Empowerment of women must be supported.

Third, we must accelerate agricultural productivity. Agriculture is the lifeblood of the economy in low-income developing countries. In those countries, it provides up to three-quarters of all employment and half of all incomes. There are very strong links between agricultural productivity increases and broad-based economic growth in the rest of the economy. Agriculture is an engine of growth in low-income developing countries. National and international agricultural research systems must be mobilised to develop improved technologies focused on developing countries, and extension systems must be strengthened to disseminate the improved technologies and techniques. Low-income countries currently spend less than 0.5 per cent of the value of agricultural production on agricultural research compared to 2 per cent spent on agricultural research in middle and high-income countries. An increase of agricultural research expenditures in low-income countries to at least 1 per cent of the value of a agricultural output is urgently need, with a longer term target of 2 per cent. National agricultural research must be supported by a vibrant international agricultural research system that undertakes research with large international benefit applicable across boundaries. Current investments in international agricultural research are grossly inadequate to provide the support needed by developing countries. It is of critical importance that agricultural research result in reduced unit costs of production. Such cost reductions will make food economically accessible to low-income consumers, and permit producer incomes to increase. To assure relevance of research and appropriate distribution of responsibilities, interactions between public sector agricultural research systems, farmers, private enterprises, and NGOs must be strengthened.

Fourth, we must assure sustainability in agricultural production and sound management of natural resources. Farmers, local communities, and governments must be encouraged to establish and enforce systems of rights to use and manage natural resources, to improve the way water is allocated and used, to reverse land degradation where it has occurred, to reduce the use of chemical pesticides and promote integrated pest management programs, and to implement integrated soil fertility programs in areas with low soil fertility. Local control over natural resources must be strengthened and local capacity for organisation and management improved. Investments in less-favored geographical areas, that is, areas with agricultural potential, irregular rainfall patterns, and fragile soils must be expanded. Most poor people in developing countries reside in rural areas, and most rural poor reside in less-favoured areas. Yet, most investments, including agricultural research investments, still focus on the more-favoured areas. If we are serious about reducing poverty and protecting the natural resource base, the balance between the less-favoured and more-favoured areas must be redressed.

Fifth, we must reduce food-marketing costs in low-income developing countries. The cost of bringing food from the producer to the consumer is very high in many of these countries. Efficient, effective, and low-cost agricultural markets must be developed in order to bring these costs down. Inefficient state-run firms in agricultural in-put markets must be phased out; investment in developing and maintaining infrastructure, especially in rural areas, must be forthcoming; policies and institutions that favour large-scale, capital-intensive market agents over small-scale, labour-intensive ones must be removed; development of small-scale credit and savings institutions must be facilitated, and technical assistance to create or strengthen small-scale, labour-intensive competitive rural enterprises must be provided.

Sixth, we must expand and realign international development assistance. Many years ago, industrialised countries had agreed to allocate at least 0.7 per cent of the gross national product (GNP) to international assistance. Most countries have not reached or do not maintain this target. No only must the industrialised countries increase international development assistance to reach the 0.7 per cent target, but they must realign it to low-income developing countries. Also contrary to the middle-and higher-income developing countries, the poorest countries are not able to gain access to capital from the rapidly expanding international commercial capital market. Developing countries in turn must seek measures to diversify sources of external funding, stem capital flight; and improve the effectiveness of the aid they receive.

21

India's Food Challenge

Is India's population growing disproportionately to its food supply? Will famine once again hit millions of people? Most agriculture experts agree that a Malthusian crisis is not likely to occur in the near term. The reason; the overall food situation in India has been characterised by a large increase in regional output since the famine-ravaged 1960s.

At that time, the food situation was described as "desperate" in India. Famine had plagued India's Bihar state in the sixties. International food specialists predicted further famine because food production looked as if it would lag for behind population growth. Instead, average crop yields per acre soared, thanks to the introduction of high-yielding varieties of rice and wheat and to expanded irrigation and chemical fertilizer use. It has been called the "green revolution".

Double Role of Irrigation

The keys to the higher food production have been irrigation, the adoption of high-yielding varieties (HYVs) of foodgrains and the increased use of modern inputs such as fertilizers. Irrigation has played a double role, it has not only helped raise yields through synergistic interaction with HYVS and fertilizers, but has also contributed to considerable increases in harvested area by enabling higher cropping intensity.

Still, there are ominous clouds on Indian food horizon. In light of the region's high population growth, increased urban sprawl and rampant environmental degradation, there are signs that hunger problems could loom unless action is taken by Indians and international development agencies.

Shrinking Base

The favourable food supply situation is likely to disappear within the next decade, due to a shrinking resource base, The earlier decades had witnessed a natural resources based growth strategy as there was adequate land and water resources for development. But this is fast disappearing due to urbanisation, industrialisation and ecological degradation. We should also remember that about 50 per cent of food production is from rainfed lands and a few years of drought could alter the food security which we now enjoy. The high costs of irrigation and land development, coupled with low commodity prices, are also hampering required investments and these effects will be seen in the next decade.

"By the year 2030, India will have to produce 60 per cent more rice with much fewer resources. Clearly, there will be a major challenge for scientists and policy-makers to meet the increased food demand. India's population is growing 2 per cent a year, making the challenges for regional food security a daunting task.

The solution for meeting future food demand will be breakthroughs in science and technology since yield levels have reached a plateau and are even showing signs of decline. The possibilities through biotechnology and genetic engineering are exciting and can herald another "green revolution". This is the only hope for avoiding the Malthusian dilemma.

In gauging the region's population-food squeeze, it is useful to look first at its swelling population. India—the world's second populous region contains several states with high population growth rates.

Ironic Problem

Rapid population growth dilutes and impedes economic development. An increase in the population base puts greater pressure on finite resources, both financial and natural, and, in the context, worsening of income distribution, increased poverty incidence and environmental degradation.

Moreover, there is the ironic problem, that although rapid population growth increases poverty, poverty encourages larger families through its impact on access to education and decreased prospects for child survival.

If population growth is uncontrolled, the economic and social consequences are:

- ecological imbalance, with greater pressure on natural resources.
- increased urban crowding, with increases in demand for municipal services and infrastructure.
- a more unequal income distribution, particularly as labour supply outpaces job creation.
- signs of mass poverty, including high infant and child mortality rates, high levels of child malnutrition and hunger, poor school performance, unemployment and underemployment.

Bleak Prospects

Existing population growth rates is unsustainable, even for the relatively near future. Unless population growth rate is kept within manageable limits, the prospects for creating acceptable standards of living for low-income groups in India will be bleak.

The Indian population is growing more rapidly than ever before and will continue to do so for at least four decades. Indeed, without major technological breakthroughs and changes in patterns of consumption, even the most optimistic population growth projections are likely to be accompanied by increase in poverty, hunger and environmental degradation.

Whether we look at population, the environment or development, the next 10 years will be critical for our future, The decisions we make or don't take will widen or narrow our options for a century to come. They could decide the fate of the earth as a home for human beings.

Less Food Security in the South

Combating hunger and poverty is the central point of Bread for the world' s mandate. In our view, that is not so much about the quantity of food produced in the world. On the one hand, it's about its fair distribution and, on the other, the access of poor people to chances of jobs. Put another way, it's to do with access to purchasing power. In the case of agriculture, that is bound up with the question of how food is produced. Whether the technologies applied maximize employment or replace work with capital.

"Hunger Though Surplus"

The question of production, employment and distribution are tied closely tc the general conditions for development. It is certainly not exclusively external economic conditions, which account for hunger and under-development. Structural deficits, political conditions and wrong policies in Third World countries have become increasingly clear. However, it can still be noted that global economic framework conditions remain enormously important for the development of agriculture in the Third World.

Twenty years ago, Bread for the world publicly expounded the thesis "Hunger through surplus" and had to take much criticism for it—above all from agro-economists. But since then the contradiction between the ever-growing mountains of agricultural surpluses in the northern hemisphere and the increasing dependence on food imports of the South has become ever more apparent. Out of 120 poor developing countries, 107 today are net importers of food.

The North's surpluses of dairy products, grain, beef and sugar—which because of their production costs are exorbitantly expensive—thrust their way on to world market and destroy local supply systems (which are cheap because of subsidies), regional trade flows, and the sales possibilities of potential Third World agro-exporters. Thus, the surpluses contribute to the situation that in many developing countries a policy of neglecting local agriculture can be continued with impurity.

Initially, the promise to work on the yawning gap between hunger and surplus in the world was upfront on WTO agenda. But the pattern of explanation was well simplified. It said that surpluses arose only in those countries, which supported their agriculture positively and, in fact, partly excessively. And that agricultural deficiencies in countries of the South were caused mainly by deprivation of resources and capital. However, the concept of not only reducing neglect of agriculture in the South but also its oversubsidising in the North to a sensible degree and thereby eliminating their distortions of world markets had a great intellectual attraction. At any rate, it promised more justice in agriculture.

Subsidies Can Make Sense

To avoid misunderstandings, we have nothing against the support of agriculture in Europe. Above all not when it is done for social, ecological or agriculturally beneficial reasons.

On the contrary, agriculture's important role for food security, the sustainable handling of natural resources, the settlement of rural areas, and the social function of family farms justify a special position for it is economic life, including protection and support.

But that must not be carried so far that surpluses are produced with the help of dubious production methods and then dumped on the world market at markedly less than cost price, causing incalculable damage in the poor countries. On the other hand, purposeful promotion of rural development is a prerequisite and model for greater self-sufficiency worldwide, especially in Third World countries.

Complementary Functions 0f World Markets

The poor countries of the South have no alternative than to become self-sufficient in food. The World markets can at best assume complementary functions. The countries would take indeterminable risks if they integrated themselves completely in the world markets, and thereby wanted to make themselves dependent upon global agro-markets. These are and will remain extremely unreliable factors that are conditioned by enormous fluctuations in prices and quantities, the powerful, and in many cases obscure, influences of multinational concerns, the manifold political interventions in the agricultural scene in most countries, and the dangers of social and ecological dumping.

But when we now look at the results of the WTO, we are disappointed. The development question and the balancing of hunger and surplus are finally no longer on the agenda. Programmes to increase food production in the poor countries were not the priority of the negotiations. The liberalisation of agro-policies in the developing countries would have meant making the disadvantaging of their farmers the subject of international negotiations. That did not happen.

On the contrary, the concepts developed with an eye on the reform of agricultural policy in the North, which target the reduction of the support level, are to be transferred to the South without questions. To be sure, there are a whole number of exemptions for the poorest developing countries. But the WTO results have also set the trend there, namely the dismantlement of subsides. We cannot understand how such a thing can be demanded as a policy programme, especially for Africa. Support for African agriculture is largely absent, i.e. there is absolutely nothing to dismantle. That's why many international conferences repeatedly emphasise the need for the countries to achieve a greater degree of self-sufficiency in food by stronger support of their agriculture.

Agro-Dumping

Certainly, some changes have been made in the North's agro policy system, which will also have positive impacts on world agricultural markets. However, also here we must express our disappointment. Agricultural dumping will continue. The only difference will be the new policy instrument of direct transfer of income instead of subsidised grain prices. The opening of markets in future will hardly go beyond the current preference conditions.

The entire set of W.T.O. agreements, however, bears the imprint of the two agricultural superpowers, the USA and the European Union, which make mutual concessions and coordinate their agricultural policies. But one hears nothing about the target of freeing the world agricultural market from unnecessary distortions and ensuring justice. The intention of the agro-superpowers was solely to defend their global market shares.

The development aid agencies cannot close their eyes to these problems. On the contrary, in future they must make very much greater effort in suggesting better goals, programmes and instruments which are capable of forming a policy that can then be included in the agenda of the next rounds of negotiations. We may perhaps have slept a bit through the past WTO talks. Therefore it is even more important that we get very much more involved from now on.

23

Genetic Diversity and Food Security

Maintaining a diversity of crops and varieties is a key to survival for millions of farmers living on impoverished land. For thousands of years, farmers have used the genetic variation in wild and cultivated plants to develop their crops and raise new breeds of live stock. Genetic diversity gives species the ability to adapt to changing environments, including new pests and diseases and new climatic conditions. Plant genetic resources—that component of genetic diversity of actual or potential use to humanity—provide the raw material for breeding new varieties of crops. These, in turn, provide a basis for more productive and resilient production systems that are better able to cope with such stresses as drought or overgrazing and can reduce the potential for soil erosion. The use of genetic diversity—on-farm, through field experimentation or in sophisticated gene transfer procedures—remains arguably the best route so securing our food and that of our children.

Although science has made enormous strides in improving the world's ability to feed itself over the past three decades, we cannot afford to rest idle. Nearly 800 million people in the developing world do not have enough to eat. In these regions, the rural poor represent about 73 per cent of the people living in poverty. They often live in marginal or unsuitable farming areas, such as zones with saline soils, and conditions, or degraded or hilly areas. Often isolated from other farms and far from urban areas, many poor farmers have barely benefited from agricultural developments elsewhere. In many cases they do no have access to commercially bred high yielding crop varieties. Diversity flourishes and remains important under such conditions.

Selections and Breeding

Poor farmers are well aware of the relationship between the stability and sustainability of crops and crop varieties on their lands. Their management and use of a diverse range of plants has often helped them to survive under the most difficult conditions. By growing a range of different crops, farmers have a better chance of meeting their needs. These might be crops that mature at different times or that can be easily stored to help to ensure a stable food supply throughout the year. They may also help farmers provide a nutritionally balance diet for their families, exploit different environment niches that exist on their land, or diversity their income sources.

Importantly, the genetic diversity contained in different varieties provides farmers with options to develop, through selection and breeding, new and more productive crops that are resistant to pests and diseases. The result may be a vast range of local varieties of crops grown by farmers in any one area.

Not respecting diversity can incur high costs: in 18th century Ireland, where potatoes were the only significant source of food for about one third of the population, farmers came to rely almost entirely on one very fertile and productive variety, which proved susceptible to the devastating potato blight fungus. The resulting famine caused the death or emigration of more than 20 per cent of the population.

The value of diversity goes well beyond its ability to support stable production systems in marginal environments. As the world's human popualtion rises, environmental problems (desertification, deforestation, erosion etc.) are intensifying, Climate change, particularly global warming, could bring about drastic changes in the location of the world's agro-ecological zones. Farmers will require new crop varieties capable of producing under diverse conditions, without adding ever-increasing amounts of fertilizers and other agro-chemicals. Because of the limited scope for growth in the world's cultivated areas, each new generation of varieties will have to be more productive than its predecessors.

Much has been written about the use of genetic engineering in plant breeding. Modern molecular techniques can be used to transfer genes from one living organism to another or to change the genetic material within to produce more desirable traits. Genetic Engineering has enormous potential to help solve problems that have proved intractable using conventional breeding approaches, such as developing crop varieties with in-built resistance to keep pests and diseases and tolerance to stresses such as drought. However, the possible impact of these techniques, particularly on human health and the environment, is giving rise to fierce worldwide debate.

Take the case of banana and its close relative plantain, two of the developing world's most important crops. Their improvement is hindered by the sterility of most cultivars, a problem that can be addressed through genetic engineering. It is now possible to transfer gene constructs, such as those associated with disease resistance, directly into varieties with other desirable characteristics, drastically reducing the need for pesticides.

Today, research on genetic engineering is focussed on the development of commercial vrieties of the world's major crops of interest to industrialised farmers. Many of the staple crops of importance to poor farmers in developing countries, such as cassava, bananas, beans and yams, have received relatively little attention. This situation is likely to continue as plant breeding is increasingly privatised and biotechnology becomes the fast-growing province of private industry. Meanwhile, the high costs of the new technologies are quickly exceeding the capacity of many, if not most, public research institutions—both in developing and developed countries—to support them. Thus, for the time being, increasing agriculture's role in the development of the world's poor is likely to continue to depend on the identification, maintenance and use of genetic diversity.

24

Population Growth and Cropland

Since mid-century, global population has grown much faster than the cropland area. The trend is likely to continue in the next century, dropping cropland per person to historically low levels. The ever smaller per capita cropland bases will make food self-sufficiency impossible for many countries, and will test the capacity of international markets to meet a growing demand for imported food.

For millennia, farmers satisfied rising food demand by bringing new land under the plow. But by mid-century cropland expansion could no longer meet the food needs of an increasingly populous and prosperous world. The 10,000 year era of steady expansion was over, and a new era began that stressed raising land productivity. As this high-yielding era shows signs of faltering, concern over the shrinking supply of cropland per person looms ever larger.

Since mid-century, grain area—which serves as a proxy for cropland in general—has increased by some 19 per cent, but global population has grown 132 per cent, seven times faster. Largely as a result, grain area per person has fallen by half since 1950, from 0.24 to 0.12 hectares. Assuming that grain area remains constant, grain area per person will fall to 0.07 hectares by 2050. In crowded industrial countries such as Japan, Taiwan, and South Korea, grain area per capita today is smaller than the area of a tennis court.

As grain area per person falls, more and more nations risk losing the capacity to feed themselves. Having already seen per capita grain area shrink by 40-50 per cent between 1960 and 1998, Pakistan, Nigeria, Ethiopia, and Iran can expect a further 60-70 per cent loss by 2050—a conservative projection that assumes no further losses of agricultural land. The result will be four countries with a combined population of more than 1 billion whose grain area per person will be only 300-600 square metres, less than a quarter of the area in 1950.

The historical record suggests that such a small area per person will send a substantial share of a country's people to world markets for their food. Consider the experience of six countries in East Asia whose per capita grain area currently ranges from 200 to 600 square metres per person. Sri Lanka relies on imports for more than a third of its grain, while Japan, Thiwan, South Korea, and Malaysia buy more than 70 per cent of their grain from abroad. North Koera is the only one of the six that does not import heavily (it gets less than 20 per cent of its grain requirements from abroad), but its population is poorly fed-indeed, on the verge of starvation.

The concern is that population growth will push many nations—not just the four fastest-growing ones—below the 600-square metre-threshold in coming decades. In Asia alone, where grain area per person stands at 800 square metres, 16 countries are poised to cross this threshold by 2050, and many of them much sooner. As this process unfolds, the number of people who will turn to foreign markets for their food will likely jump sharply. These countries will find an increasingly tight international grain market, with nations from the Middle East, North Africa, and other regions already buying a third or more of their grain overseas.

In addition to per capita losses, population growth can lead to degradation of cropland, reducing its productivity or even eliminating it from production. As a country's population density increases and good farmland becomes scarce, poor farmers are forced onto ecologically vulnerable land such as hillsides and tropical forest. In the Philippines, for example, hillside agriculture accounted for only 10 per cent of all agricultural land in 1960, but 30 per cent in 1987. Because it is highly erodible, hillside land is easily damaged; worldwide, some 160 million hectares of hillside farmland—11 per cent of cropland—were characterised in 1989 as "severely eroded." Similarly, population pressure can force peasants to overfarm the poor soils of tropical forests. After being cleared and farmed for a few years, these soils typically require fallow period of 20-25 years, but population pressures keep poor farmers on the same land for far longer than the soils can support, cutting fallow period to just a few years in some areas of tropical Africa and Asia.

Finally, population pressures on a fixed base of land can result in rural landlessness. In Bangladesh, for example, landlessness among rural households rose from 35 per cent in 1960 to 53 per cent in the early 1990s. Interestingly, Bangladesh is regarded as a success in slowing population expansion, as its growth rate declined from 2.8 per cent in the late 1970s to 1.5 per cent in the early 1990s. But its success came too late to prevent the increase in rural landlessness, highlighting the need to work sooner, rather than later, for population stabilisation.

25

Population Growth and Grain Production

The relationship between the growth in world population and the grain harvest has shifted over the last half-century, neatly dividing this period into two distinct eras. From 1950 to 1984, growth and the grain harvest easily exceeded that of population, raising the harvest per person from 247 kilograms to 342, a gain of 38 per cent. During the 14 years since then, growth in the grain harvest has fallen behind that of population, dropping output per person from its historic high in 1984 to an estimated 317 kilograms in 1998—a decline of 7 percent, or 0.5 per cent a year.

These global trends conceal widely divergent developments among countries, contrasts that can be seen for the world's two most populous nations: India and China. In both, grain production per person was close to 200 kilograms as recently as 1978. Since then, the figure in India has edged up slightly but still falls short of 200 kilograms, while in China production has surged since the economic reforms in 1978, with per-person output now at nearly 300 kilograms. The combination of a dramatic surge in grain production and an equally dramatic reduction in population growth has given China a large margin of safety, effectively eliminating most of its hunger and malnutrition. Meanwhile, although India has also achieved impressive gains in its harvest, these have been largely cancelled by population growth, leaving its 976 million people living close to the margin.

What has happened in China and India is the story of developing countries in general. The overwhelming majority have achieved substantial, if not dramatic, gains in their grain harvests over the last half-century. Some, such as Thailand, have combined this with a much slower growth of population, which means that agricultural gains translate into rising grain production per person. In Pakistan, by contrast, grain production per person climbed steadily for a while, but it peaked in 1981 at 186 kilograms. Since then it has been declining nearly 1 per cent a year. In effect, Pakistan's farmers are losing the battle with population growth.

The slower growth in the world grain harvest since 1984 is due to the lack of new land and to slower growth in irrigation and fertilizer use. Irrigated area per person, after expanding by 4 per cent since then as growth in the irrigated area has fallen behind that of population.

The increase in world fertiliser use has slowed dramatically since 1990, as diminishing returns to the application of additional fertilizer has stabilized use in the United States, Western Europe, and Japan and slowed annual growth in world fertilizer use from 6 per cent between 1950 and 1990 to scarcely 2 per cent in recent years.

Although Malthus was primarily concerned with the additional demand for grain generated by population growth, rising affluence is also playing a role. In a low income country such as India, grain consumption per person is less than 200 kilograms per year and diets are typically dominated by a single starchy staple-rice, for instance. With scarcely a pound of grain available a day per person, nearly all must be consumed directly, leaving little for conversion into animal protein. For the average American, on the other hand, the great bulk of the 800-kilogram daily grain consumption is taken in indirectly in the form of beef, pork, poultry, eggs, milk, cheese, ice cream, and yogurt. At the intermediate level, in a country like Italy, people consume 400 kilograms of grain a day. Future food price stability thus depends on expanding production fast enough to keep up with both population growth and rising affluence.

One question often asked is, How many people can the Earth support? This must be answered with another question, At what level of consumption? If the world grain harvest of 1.87 billion tons were expanded to 2 billion tons in the years ahead, it would support 10 billion Indians or 2.5 billion Americans. To answer the question of how many people the Earth can support, we first have to know the level of consumption we expect to live at.

Now that the frontiers of agricultural settlement have disappeared, future growth in grain production must come almost entirely from raising land productivity. Unfortunately, this is becoming more difficult. After rising at 2.1 per cent a year from 1950 to 1990, the annual increase in rainland productivity dropped to scarcely 1 per cent from 1990 to 1997. The challenge for the world's farmers is to reverse this decline at a time when cropland area per person is shrinking, the amount of irrigation water per person is dropping, and the crop yield response to additional fertilizer use is falling.

26

Population Growth and Meat Production

World meat production increased from 44 million tons almost twice as fast as population. In per capita terms, world meat production expanded from 17 kilograms in 1950 to 36 kilograms in 1997, more than doubling. Growth in meat production was originally concentrated in western industrial countries and Japan, but over the last two decades it has increased rapidly in East Asia (especially China), the Middle East, and Latin America.

When incomes begin to rise in traditional low-income societies, one of the first things people do is diversify their diets, consuming more livestock products. People everywhere appear to have an innate desire to consume at least moderate quantities of meat, perhaps reflecting our evolutionary history as hunter-gatherers.

Three types of meat—beef, pork, and poultry—account for the bulk of world consumption; mutton ranks a distant fourth. From 1950 until 1980, beef and pork production followed the same trend, but after the economic reforms in China—where pork is dominant—pork production surged ahead, climbing from 45 million tons to nearly 90 million tons in less than two decades.

Historically, growth in the world meat supply came primarily from beef and mutton, sustained by the world's rangelands. These areas, consisting mostly of land that is too arid to support crop production, cover a vast part of the planet, roughly double the cropland area. Not only do the herbs of cattle and flocks of sheep and goats provide meat and milk, but for millions of people in Africa, the Middle East, Central Asia, parts of the Indian subcontinent, and western China, they provide a livelihood. The only feasible way that this land can contribute to the world's food supply is to graze cattle, sheep, and goats on it, producing the meat and milk that directly and indirectly sustain large segment of humanity.

In recent years, beef and mutton production have levelled off at just over 60 million tons per year as the number of animals has pressed against the carrying capacity of range lands. With little unused grazing capacity left, future gains in meat production will have to come largely from feeding animals grain. At this point, the relative conversion efficiency of various animals begins to influence production trends. Producing a kilogram of beef in the feedlot requires roughly seven kilograms of grain, while a kilogram of pork requires nearly four of grain and a kilogram of poultry, just over two. As grain supplies tighten, the advantage shifts from beef to pork and even more so to poultry. This helps explain why world poultry production overtook that of beef in 1996.

Of the world grain harvest of 1.87 billion tons in 1998, an estimated 37 per cent or nearly 700 million tons—will be used to feed livestock and poultry, production milk and eggs as well as meat. This share, remarkably stable for the last decade, could go up or down depending on future grain prices.

Expanding world meat production also depends on soyabean production. If the grain fed to livestock or poultry is supplemented with a modest amount of soyabean meal (the high protein meal that is left after the oil is extracted), its conversion into meat is much more efficient. Largely as a result of this growing demand for livestock products, world soyabean production climbed from 17 million tons in 1950 to 152 million tons in 1997, a gain of ninefold.

To project the future demand for meat, we assume that the growth in meat consumption per person will slow over the next half-century, rising by one half instead of doubling, since some countries are nearing the saturation point. This, combined with the projected growth in population, would push total meat consumption from 211 million tons in 1997 to 513 million tons in 2050, a gain of 302 million tons. If we assume an average of 3 kilograms of grain per kilogram of meat produced, this would require more than 900 million tons of additional grain for feed in 2050, an amount equal to half of current world grain consumption. This would greatly intensify the competition between grain consumed directly and that consumed indirectly as animal protein, calling into question whether such gains in meat consumptions will ever materialize.

Grain fed to livestock and poultry is now the principal food reserve in the event of a world food emergency. As of 1990, the world had, in effect, three reserves in the global food system: substantial stocks of grain that could be drawn upon in the event of unexpected shortages, a large area of cropland idled under U.S. farm commodity programmes, and grain fed to animals. By 1998, world grain stocks had been depleted to one of the lowest levels on record and the cropland that was idled for half a century was returned to production. The only safety net remaining in the event of a major crop failure is the grain fed to livestock and poultry.

27

Population Growth and Oceanic Fish Catch

Form 1950 until 1988, the oceanic fish catch soared from 19 million to 88 million tons, expanding much faster than population. The per capita catch increased from less than 8 kilograms in 1950 to the historical peak of just over 17 kilograms in 1988, more than doubling since 1988, however, growth in the catch has slowed, falling behind that of population. Between 1988 and 1996, the catch per person declined to less than 16 kilograms, a drop of some 9 per cent.

This five-fold growth in the human appetite for seafood since 1950 has pushed the catch of most oceanic fisheries to their sustainable limits or beyond. Marine biologists believe that the oceans cannot sustain an annual catch of much more than 93 million tons, the current take.

As we near the end of the twentieth century, over fishing has become the rule, not the exception. Of the 15 major oceanic fisheries. 11 are in decline. The catch of Atlantic cod-long a dietary mainstay for West Europeans-has fallen by some 70 per cent since peaking in 1968. Since 1970, bluefin tuna stocks in the West Atlantic have dropped 80 per cent.

The next half-century is likely to be marked by the disappearance of some species from markets, a decline in the quality of seafood caught, higher prices, and more conflicts among countries over access to fisheries. Over the last two decades, a growing share of the catch has consisted of inferior species, some of which were not even considered edible in times past.

The growing scarcity of the species at the top of the food chain is reflected in rising prices. Poor people who once ate fish because they could not afford meat now find that meat is often less expensive than seafood. Although most price rises are moderate, some are extreme going far beyond anything we could have earlier imagined. The decline of the bluefin tuna population in the Atlantic, for instance, has occasionally pushed prices for a 300-Kilogram tuna above $80,000 at top-of-the-line sushi restaurants in Japan compete for the few of these giant fish that are available.

This growing competition for limited resources has led to ongoing conflicts among countries. The United Nations recorded more than 100 such disputes in 1997. These are evident in the cod wars between Norwegian and Icelandic ships, between Canada and Spain over turbot off Canada's eastern coast, between China and the Marshall Islands in Micronesia, between Argentina and Taiwan over Falkland island fisheries, and between Indonesia and the Philippines in the Celebes. There are "tuna wars in the northeast Atlantic, crab wars in the North Pacific, squid wars in the southwest Atlantic, salmon wars in the North Pacific, and Pollock wars in the Sea of Okhotsk." Although these disputes make it into, the world news only rarely, they are now an almost daily occurrence. Indeed, historians may record more fishery conflicts during one year in the 1990s than during the entire nineteenth century.

One of the consequences of modern fishing technologies, whether it is the use of drift nets or bottom-scouring fish-catch of unwanted species. This oceanic equivalent of clear cutting is damaging fisheries on an unprecedented scale.

With the oceans now pushed to their limits, future growth in the demand for seafood can be satisfied only by fish farming. As a result, aquaculture output has increased from 7 million tons in 1984 to an estimated 26 million tons in 1977. Most of this growth in catch is based on just a few species, such as carp, which constitute most of the aqua cultural harvest in China, and catfish, which dominates fish farming in the United States. As the world turns to fish farming to satisfy its needs, fish begin to compete with livestock and poultry for foodstuffs such as grain, soybean meal, and fish meal.

Given tha the oceanic fish catch is apparently now at or beyond its sustainable limit, it is a relatively simple matter to determine the future oceanic catch per person. With each year, this will decline by roughly the amount of population growth, drooping to 9.9. kilograms per person in 2050, a decline to little more than half the 1988 peak of 17.2 kilograms. Those of us born before 1950 have enjoyed a doubling of the seafood catch per person, while those born in recent years are likely to witness a decline of nearly one half during their lifetimes.

28

Health Care Relief in Conflict Situations:

What Can we Learn from the Food Relief Experience?

Conflicts and war occur in many of the poorest nations where populations already suffer from severs ill health. War leads to an increase in disease and to a worsening of the already fragile condition of populations. Health care itself becomes a victim of conflict. Many deaths which occur during these emergencies are not discretely related to the conflict itself but are the result of lacking access to public health services. Furthermore, conflict itself but are the result of lacking access to public health services. Furthermore, conflict contributes to the deterioration of already pre-existing structural weaknesses of the health care system. An example is the period of internal conflict in Uganda (1970-1986) when health services declined in the aftermath of the war due to the impact of foreign assistance and the planning vacuum in which the activities took place.

The Impact of Conflict on Health Care

Conflict and civil strife may lead to a major disruption of health services. This is not only a result of physical destruction but also of finding shortages since national governments increase spending on military activities. Casualties increase the demand for curative services, which can divert already limited resources from preventive care.

In the case of the Sudanese civil war a large majority of health professionals was forced to abandon rural health professionals was forced to abandon rural health services and left for urban areas or neighbouring countries in order to find new employment. Entire preventive health services such as immunisation as well as water and sanitation projects collapsed leaving the population exposed to infectious diseases and epidemics. In urban areas, the gap in public health care provision is sometimes filled with the expansion of private services. In rural areas, private sector involvement in health care is rather marginal, apart form some omission hospitals or pharmacies. Therefore the non-formal health care sector often makes a substantial contribution towards health care.

With the rise internal conflicts in Africa, more people suffer from emergency situations. This also increases the influence and impact of international donors. External assistance nowadays accounts for more than 25 per cent of government health expenditure in sub-Saharan Africa.

The size of donor involvement reflects the power of international agencies to control the policy domain. Countries in conflict or post-conflict situations are under pressure to 'rescue' their health systems and accept global policies in exchange for aid assistance and relief.

However, in the period after 1991, donor organisations tended to increase their expenditures for high profile humanitarian operations rather than ordinary development activities. This shift may reflect the increasing influence of media covering some of the conflicts. Too often, organisations intervene with ad hoc assistance without sufficient consultation at local level.

Donors' Perceptions in Designing Relief Interventions

Today, in many parts of sub-Saharan Africa development assistance has virtually collapsed and has been substituted by relief assistance. The problem is that relief intervention are based on a Western construction of reality, reflecting what is desirable and necessary in times of conflict. Most interventions therefore stress physical and material needs, presuming that the social aspect of food and health is not an immediate issue to address.

The question which arises here is on who's views and perceptions these needs are based? While donors interest may be guided from the perspective of ill-health, the recipient government may be concerned with the collapse of the economy. However, any intervention needs to take into account that local knowledge and practices are shaped by state interests as well as power relationships. The common belief that health care systems always collapse due to conflict is sometimes mistaken, considering the fact that today's internal conflicts are often fragmented, conflicts do not necessarily result in a breakdown of the health care delivery system.

Donors tend to respond with a 'package approach and developing countries ministries of health increasingly play a symbolic role. The evidence suggests that international organisation tend to create vertical programmes, which undermine national public health programmes. Foreign interventions are technically sophisticated and reorienting health are towards a more curative approach. Too little attention given to strengthen the health care system within its own limits, providing more appropriate technology, drugs and emphasizing the training of local health staff.

Another vital issue concerns the existence of already fragile health information systems. Agencies tend to bring their own systems which leads to further fragmentation. The local perspective on what are the 'basic needs' in physical and social health are usually not considered. Health relief interventions do not recognize the potential of the communities and the non-formal health sector such as healers and traditional midwifes in supporting and maintaining health care sector presents a substantial contribution towards health. It is not the question between choosing either allopathic or traditional services, it is more the decision which kind of illness will be best treated by which practitioner. There is a need in further exploring the role of this sector particularly since this is sometimes the only service available for certain populations.

Responding to Local Needs

More community-based public health intervention could

be vital to reduce mortality and morbidity. For example in Somalia during the 1992 war and famine high mortality rates due to measles and diarrhoea could have been prevented by involving the communities in primary health care activities such as immunisation and nutrition improvement.

In the African context Tigray is an example where health services had been sustained and partially expanded during the civil war against the Ethiopian government. Local government structures called baitos promoting social and economic development. Baitos encouraged communities to establish revolving funds for drugs and medical equipment. It actually functioned as early type of community financing system

As mentioned above, the challenge in changing health care relief strategies is to overcome the approach of short-term interventions, particularly in changing conflict environment where conflicts are complex and interruptions are no longer short-term.

Therefore interventions need to be linked with the process of conflict resolution to avoid health care or food aid being used by politically dominant groups.

Food Relief in Conflict Situations

Food interventions have both a survival and a production function. For example, food-for-work may be part of an income programme or food aid can be magnetised to generate local currency. However, food aids have to be seen beyond the objective to fulfill nutritional goals, it also defines relationships between social groups in regard to food accessibility and how food is shared. Food aid is aiming to meet people's basic food requirements and minimising risk and severity of disease by complementing services such as basic health care.

In more stable political conditions where free food aid is given it presents an income transfer by releasing income, which normally is spent on food. However, in conflict situations food relief frequently becomes part of the dynamics of conflict such in the case of Sudan where it is used to sustain the struggle between the North and the South without resolving it. Furthermore, the military attack food supplies in the fight against rebels who depend on the support from the communities.

Health is also a matter of food security. When food insecurity coincides with conflict situations, health and survival are threatened. Food security provided some concepts on how and why vulnerable households manage to survive in periods of hardship (coping strategies).

Coping Strategies in African Trouble Zones

Today, most conflicts in Africa such as the ones in the Great Lake Region, Angola or Congo cause major problems of food insecurity. They are linked to the civil wars which produce substantial social disruption as a result of massive population movements. The analysis of coping strategies showed that household respond to these conflict situation by eating less, selling livestock and land, or trying to find new sources of income.

In some emergency situations, however such coping mechanisms may fall. In the case of the war in Mozambique food aid was vital since coping strategies were limited and people had to sell all their assets, which was particular, true for internationally displaced persons and refugees.

It has been argued that food relief bypasses local structures in favour of those qualifying on a nutrition status criterion, decided by international organisation, or it may attract populations to refugee camps to receive free food rations and thereby undermines local production. In the case of Rwanda food aid was targeted at the internally displaced and left out the local population. This can be due to donor bias in needs assessment.

Food scarcity is not always so result of civil war but its creation may be rather a political objective. An example is food relief manipulated by local elites and the military like in the case of Sudan. It can be summarised that generally relief operations often bear the risk of fueling the process of instability and violence rather that helping to contain the situation.

Lessons from Food Relief for the Health Sector?

Through the experience of food relief in recent civil wars such as Sudan, Somalia, Mozambique etc., there has been an increasing awareness of the economic and political context in which operations takes place. Like food relief, health care is a political tool, which can, if not properly targeted, undermine peoples access to health care services. While food production is linked to food security, it is more difficult to identify factors leading to self-sufficiency in health care.

As mentioned above, food aid is aiming to insure survival. It also has an economic aspect, protecting household assets. Health care relief is targeted to assure immediate physical survival based on the importance of social health. Unfortunately, curative interventions hardly consider the socio-cultural dimension of health. Therefore it would be beneficial if health care interventions consider local norms and traditions. Interventions should be compatible and complement local health programmes. The emphasis should be on strengthening formal and non-formal health institutions both in service provision and training.

In food relief, distribution and needs assessment identification are controversial issues for discussion. While the programme design is shaped by donor's perceptions, the actual programmes are influenced by the priorities of some powerful leaders as well as the socio-economic and political context.

Health care interventions need to analyses these issues in the context of economic and political systems in order to identify the most vulnerable groups, for example populations living in areas which are more, operations require a stronger involvement of communities both as users and active participants carry out and maintain public health programmes.

There is a need for a new concept to be designed, which applies, to chronic emergencies. In the absence of a policy framework, guidelines need to be developed in order to overcome the inconsistency in planning and implementation. Donors need to change their assumptions on which they plan their health relief responses. A starting point in improving the efficiency of these operations is to provide institutional support to local authorities and organisations and involve them in the planning and implementation of programmes.

Bibliography

Aggarwal A, Patenting Gene Fragments, Economic and Political Wekkly, May, 1993.

Aggarwal J.C., and Chowdhry K.N., Dunkel Proposals, Volume I & II Shipra Publications, New Delhi-1994.

Agha Zafar, "Damming Dukel", India Today, April 15, 1994.

Bhagwati J.N., Multi-lateralism at Risk: the GATT is Dead, Long Live the GATT, The World Economy, June, 1990.

Bharati Vivek, "GATT finds India's Exports Outpacing", Economic Times, April 24, 1994.

Bharati Vivek, "Degrees of Freedom", Economic Times, January 6, 1994.

Bhattacharya A.K.,"India to Lead Global Strategy to Free Trade from Social Issues", Economic Times, April 13, 1994.

Bijlani SK What does GATT Mean for India, Doaba House Publishers, New Delhi, 1995

Chakrabarty, Gargi "Packing Up the Threads" Business Standard, August 30, 1997 P.12

Chemanant Parkay, Sustainable Advantage, "Harvard Business Review "Sept./Oct., 1988,

Dear Dorff A.V., Should Patent Protection be Extended to all Developing Countries, The World Economy, December 13, 1990.

Debroy Bibek and Jaspreet Bindra, "GATT India and Export Subsidies",

Economic Times, Jan, 15,1994.

Export Import Bank of India, The Uruguay Round Agreement Implications for Indian Exports, Occasional Paper No. 28, Bombay,1994.

Falk Richard The Challenge of Globalisation and the Emergence of Global Civil Society, RGICS October, 1993.

"Final Act", Economic Times, April 18, 1994

Fredie A. Mehta, GATT Globalisation and India. The Sunday Observer, April 24-30, 1994.

Ganesan A.V., The GATT Uruguay Round Opportunities and Challenges, RGICS, New Delhi,1994

Geneva Agenices Report, WTO Operations to Begin from January 1, 1995, December 8, 1994

Ghoi Nita, "GATT, NAFTA and all that", Economic Times., 15 December 93.

Hoekman B.M. Safeguard Provisions and International Trade Agreements Involving Services, The World Economy, Vol. 16., January, 1993.

International Monetary Fund, International Trade Policies the Uruguay Round and Beyond, 1994.

International Trade Statistic Year Book, Data Base, 1994.

Jackson J.H. Restructuring the GATT System, Royal Institute of International Affairs and Printer Publishers, London, 1990.

Jha Prem Shankar, "Dunkel Draft. The Brighter side". Economic Times, December 25, 1993.

Kainth Gursharan Singh, Export Potential of Indian Agriculture, Regency Publications New Delhi, 1996.

Mathrani L. Sheila, "WTO Ruling Victiory for Multi-lateralism" Economic Times, April 8, 1998.

Nullis Clare, "Watershed Financial Services Pact", Economic Times, December 14,1997.

Onkvisit Sak and Shaw J. John, International Marketing, Analysis and Strategy,MC. Millan Publications, Sydney, 1996.

"Opportunity Not Threat", Economic Times, February 22, 1994.

Plat Raghu, Documentary Letter of Credit and Collection, Viskion Books, New Delhi, 1996.

Raghavan Chakravarthi, "Uruguay Round and Rich Countries". The Tribune, September 27, 1994.

Index

L

M

N

O

P

R